True unsolicited comments from readers like you:

"I have read and re-read *The Natural Way* and feel expanded and open-hearted with each reading. I'll gladly share this with others as it has greatly enhanced my life. Thank you for this precious gift of joy and happiness."
—*AW, reader*

"This is so clarifying, so clearing, it's just incredible. It's just beautiful. Thank you."
—*LR, teacher*

"The depth and breadth of *The Natural Way* are wonderful. It covers so many deep issues with love, caring and kindness. It invites the reader to...explore, experience and express the possibilities of being happy. Thanks so much."
—*CM, researcher*

"A great job with an incredibly important lesson in the secret of happiness."
—*MG, executive*

"I really love it. I'm very happy. I really am finding it so beautiful. Incredible reminders for being love, being peace. Great, great job! It's really right on."
—*RB, marketer*

"What a sweet surprise!...Elegant and heartful."
—*EO, editor*

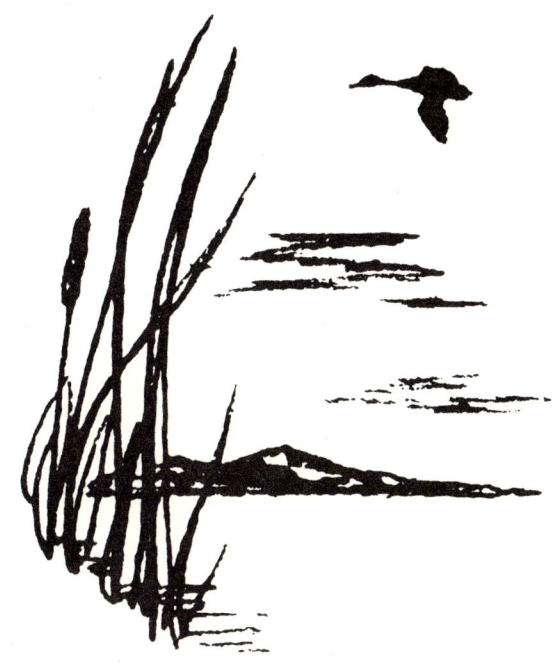

The Natural Way
AN INQUIRY INTO HAPPINESS

James Sloman

1st edition.

© 1999 by James Sloman
Project Manager: JoAnne Munley
Cover drawing by Tonia Weeks
Edited by Rebecca Bell

All rights reserved.

This book is educational.
Before making any changes in lifestyle, it is wisdom to consult an experienced advisor familiar with your personal situation.

Any OceanBlue product,
including this one, can be ordered by calling:

(800) 838-7360 (US)

(707) 838-6200 (abroad)

OceanBlue Publishing
98 Main Street
Tiburon, CA 94920

www.ocean-blue.com

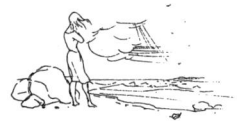

Part 1—Happiness

1. Letting Be. 11
2. Light. 16
3. Nurturing. 23
4. Mirroring 29
5. Kindness 36
6. Love 43
7. Love II. 47

Part 2—Vitality

8. True State. 55
9. Toxification 59
10. Plants 65
11. Plants II. 70
12. Living Foods. 77
13. Detoxing 83
14. Detoxing II 89
15. Well-being. 94
16. Trusting 100

Part 3—Freedom

17. Generosity............111
18. Hindrances.............116
19. Undoing................120
20. Breath.................127
21. Light..................135
22. Insight................142
23. Mystery................149

Part 4—Serenity

24. Duality................161
25. Space..................165
26. Reflections............169
27. The Voice..............174
28. Uncreation.............180
29. Choiceless.............185
30. Abundance..............189
31. Abundance II...........193
32. Four Notions...........198

Conclusion

33. The Natural Way........207

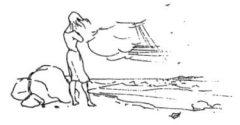

This book is an attempt to show the connection between happiness and what Lao-Tzu (and other great teachers) have called "the natural way." He said:

"The natural way is stillness."
"Rejoice in the way things are."
"Let things take their natural course."

What good can that do? And whatever does it have to do with our happiness?

Let's take a look—

PART 1
Happiness

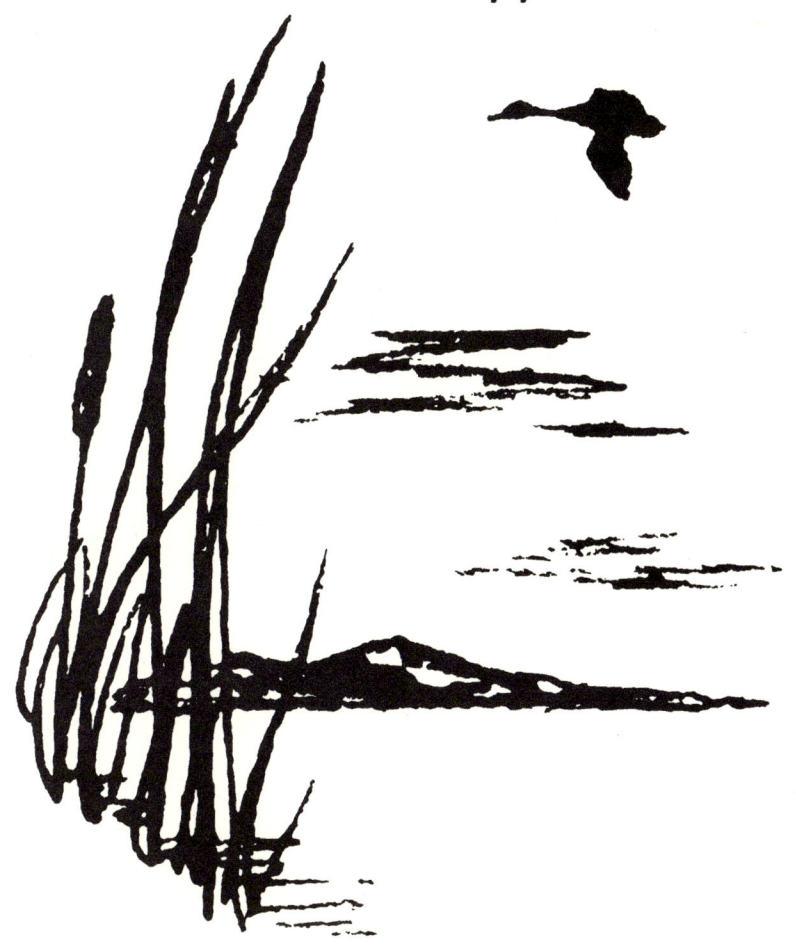

CHAPTER 1

LETTING BE

Hello to you!

Here's the deal, as far as I can tell:

We all want to be happy. And we are sometimes. But then other times we're not. And when we're not, we wonder, why aren't we happy all the time? Why does there have to be suffering?

Some very great beings have pondered that very question, including Jesus and the Buddha and Lao-Tzu and the Dalai Lama and Ramana Maharshi and Byron Katie and many others.

It seems that each of these people made a discovery and they were trying to communicate about what they discovered. I think each of them basically discovered the same thing, but because they were different people living at different times in different societies it all came out sounding different.

Here's what I sense they discovered:

That *all of our suffering arises from our disagreements with Reality.*

Now right away an objection arises, which is one I had myself for a long time. And it's this:

If I don't have some resistance to the way things are, then how can anything ever improve?

But maybe a different metaphor is called for:

Imagine that you're a gardener, and you've planted a seed in the ground. Now is there anything wrong with that seed? No, of course not. It's perfect just the way it is. Nevertheless, there's a place for watering it, for nurturing it each day.

Maybe this world is like that. Maybe the world is perfect just the way it is—and there's a place for nurturing it, too.

"Resist not evil," Jesus said to us. The "evil" part is a mistranslation, I believe. What he really meant, in my opinion, was to let go of our contractions around any part of this existence that we find unacceptable.

Why? Because to the extent that we resist anything or anybody being the way they are, we're going to hurt. We're going to suffer.

But then how will anything change?

Paradoxically, when we can let go inside of our need for anything or anybody to be different than they are, things change on their own in a mysterious way.

Because now we're nurturing that seed with love. And that perfect seed tends to grow into something else equally perfect, maybe a beautiful apple tree. It's perfect all the way through the process.

Maybe the world is that way.

My friend Byron Katie says that she's simply stopped arguing with Reality. Because she noticed that everytime she did, she felt disconnected, fearful or whatever. She didn't feel good.

And she noticed that whenever she's not arguing with Reality, she automatically feels good. Why not? Maybe we were meant to feel good and in tune. Maybe that's our natural state.

And what prevents us from being in our natural state? Maybe it's our ideas about how the world or this person or that situation or whatever should be different somehow.

Sosan, the third master of Zen, put it this way:

"The great Way is not difficult for those who cease to cherish their opinions."

I don't know about you, but I notice that my mind has all kinds of stories about how things ought to be in the future, how they should have been in the past, and so on and so forth.

The Natural Way

Apparently that's what minds do. They make up stories about how things should be or should have been, or how they ought to change or be different somehow. Or how somebody—yes, maybe even ourselves—ought to change or be different.

But as far as I can tell, everything in this Existence can't help being the way it is. It just is that way.

Can you help being the way you are? No, of course not. You're just that way. Maybe tomorrow you'll be different in some way, but right now you can't help being the way you are.

But here's the interesting thing. When somebody loves you exactly the way you are, you tend to blossom. You tend to grow. You tend to flower.

You may even leave behind some old "negative" patterns based on anger or fear or feeling hurt in some way. Some kind of contraction that you had.

But notice that it's the people who love and accept you just the way you are, who have no resistance to the way you are right now, who allow you to blossom into something more expanded.

Conversely—check this out for yourself—when you're around somebody who has a problem with you, who feels there's something wrong with you, who feels that you need to be "fixed" somehow, don't you tighten up? Resist them? Not much blossoming there.

Love is what makes the difference. The willingness

to let go of all the resistance to the way things are. And paradoxically, then they get to be different. Then that perfect seed gets to blossom into a more mature kind of existence.

Everybody I mentioned earlier, and lots of other folks that I didn't mention, mainly people we tend to think of as spiritual masters of one sort or another—here's what I think happened to them:

They fell in love with Existence.

Exactly as it is. Right down to the last grain of sand. They let go of all their stories about how it ought to be, and all their resistances to how it is.

And as soon as they did that, all their suffering stopped. Because there was no resistance anymore to cause any suffering. Then they could just hang out with this beautiful Existence and love it the way it is.

It's that very love that waters the seed and allows it to grow into something more evolved.

CHAPTER 2

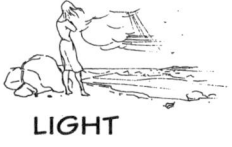

LIGHT

"Hatred never ceases by hatred. Hatred only ceases by love," the Buddha said.

Picture yourself facing a large dragon. This dragon can represent anybody or anything that you have resistance to or about deep down. Deep down, we feel they or it should be different.

And we have a story about this dragon. This dragon is wrong, should not have done what they did, should not be the way they are, should not have treated me or us or my nation or my religion or my sex or whatever that way.

Whatever happened should not have happened. It was wrong to have happened that way. It shouldn't be that way now. It or they are wrong.

This is our suffering.

The Buddha said that all suffering is caused by attachment. Attachment to what? To our stories, concepts, ideas, beliefs, to the very things that we know to be most "true."

I notice that my mind has a story about everything and everybody. Some are "good," some are "bad."

I notice that my mind makes judgments about everything. This is good, that is bad, this is beautiful, that is ugly, this is right, that is wrong, this is desirable, that is not desirable.

On and on, judging. Comparing. Deciding what's right and what's wrong. And condemning the "wrong."

The master Osho suggested a beautiful metaphor:

Picture yourself being in a darkened room. And imagine that you're walking around and you're stumbling over the furniture, because you can't see. Now you can fight with that furniture, with that darkness. But fighting with darkness becomes exhausting because darkness basically doesn't exist; it's just an absence of light.

Once you turn on the light, the problem of stumbling over the furniture disappears immediately because now you can see. The problem disappears as a by-product of more light being in the situation. You don't need to "defeat" the furniture.

Our problems are like this. When we relax into letting things be the way they are, into being friends with

The Natural Way

Existence, something miraculous happens. That little seed of beauty that was there starts growing now.

For instance, suppose we're having a problem with someone. We don't like the way they've behaved. We're irritated, disappointed or fearful of them.

Now suppose we were to just let go of our story about how they ought to be. We just relax it, like letting a closed fist open.

What then? Do we let that person walk all over us? Do we take back the person we broke up with? Do we let somebody who's harming us continue to do so? Do we keep putting up with this behavior pattern?

No, it doesn't mean that. But what we'll do can't be predicted either, because now our acts won't come from a rule or a story; they'll come from a different perspective. What we do will look like whatever it looks like, but now it will come from our intuitive heart guidance, the guidance that operates below the realm of stories and tends to produce more harmonious and magical results.

Conversely, asking "negative" types of questions— What's wrong with this person? situation? world? etc.— tends not to lead to the best kinds of outcomes, because they focus our attention on what we don't want or like, thus actually reinforcing it.

However we answer or deal with such questions, we're still putting our attention on what's wrong and thus "growing" that.

Because wherever we put our attention flourishes and grows in our life. Whatever we put our thought and feeling on becomes more real for us, and then we have to deal with it more often.

Peter Drucker, the management guru, advised businesses to "starve the problem, feed the opportunity."

Not that we ignore the problem, whatever it is, but that we start transferring more of our attention to whatever opportunity exists in the situation.

How do we find that opportunity? Tony Robbins, the neurolinguistic mentor, advises asking ourselves questions to direct our attention. Questions such as:

What am I happy about?
What am I proud of?
What am I grateful for?
What am I committed to?

Asking such questions shifts our attention to something more fruitful.

He then advises addressing the problem itself and asking questions such as these:

What's great about this?
How can I use this?

It's a way of focusing attention on the opportunity. And then the opportunity grows, because we've changed the agenda. We're putting our attention on something new, the opportunity, and that grows instead.

Let's take an example.

The Natural Way

When I was a boy my father decided it would save electricity if the lights were turned out whenever we left a room. So he suggested to me that I do that. And here's what happened:

When I did turn out the lights, it was ignored. It was expected. But when I didn't, my Dad would remind me that I hadn't turned out the lights, sometimes with increasing irritation that I wasn't "getting it."

My father had a very good heart and his intention was well-meaning. But he didn't understand the principle involved, and neither did I.

Rationally, that approach makes sense, doesn't it? You tell someone what they're doing wrong, as often as necessary, and then they correct it and do the "right" thing instead.

Unfortunately, it doesn't work very well that way. In this example, because I was frequently being negatively reinforced and almost never positively reinforced, I never did learn to turn out the lights when leaving a room.

I would make resolutions about it, I would try my best, but I still failed to do it again and again. And each time it was pointed out to me. I was a "failure" at it. Because of that and similar issues, the relationship between my Dad and I fared poorly as well.

It took me about 45-50 years of life to really begin to understand the simple principle that my father could have used. All he needed to do was the exact opposite—

Pt 1—Happiness

that is, appreciate me when I did turn out the lights and just ignore it when I didn't.

Then he would have been feeding the opportunity, starving the problem. He would have been watering—with his attention—what he did want rather than what he didn't. The results would have been vastly different.

One time I watched a father push his daughter on a swing. And what I noticed that day was this: That he always pushed the swing in the direction it was already going. When the swing was going the "opposite" way, the father just ignored that. Then when the swing was going in the "fruitful" direction again, the father would reinforce that.

When I got my cat Nicky about eight years ago, he was really a handful. Apparently he had been misused by his previous owners, because if you got within about four feet of him he would put up his claws and bare his fangs and hiss and spit. He was a pretty scared and angry and neurotic cat.

Anyway, when he did that I would just ignore it. I would just go about my business and leave him alone. But whenever he would let me get a little bit closer to him, perhaps by accident, I would give him a little snack immediately.

As time went on and he let me pet him, I would pet him and show him I loved him as much as possible, and just ignore any hostile behavior.

The Natural Way

What happened is that he eventually relaxed and turned into this beautiful animal with a wonderful personality. He still has a bit of an "edge" to him until he gets to know somebody, but once he gets to know them a little bit, he's a relaxed, affectionate cat. He's enjoying his life.

By appreciating the beautiful Being latent in Nicky and reinforcing that, he became more of his natural self. We all have that beautiful Being inside of us because we all partake of Existence.

When we look for the beautiful seed in any situation and water that with our attention and our love, then that seed starts to grow into its natural potential, which is harmony, love, joy, creativity, spontaneity, and so on—the natural Self of the situation or person.

CHAPTER 3

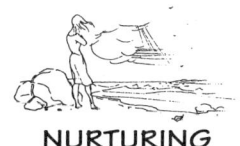
NURTURING

How do we find that Self or that natural seed of the situation? We look for it. As Jesus said, we get what we ask for, we find what we're looking for. So we have the intention to find it.

And then we "jump out of the system," as hakomi founder Ron Kurtz advised. We look at it all in a new way that doesn't remain boxed in by the old way.

Perhaps the most fundamental way to do that, to shift our perspective in a situation, is to begin to release the stories we have about it, to release our resistance to whatever is there, to cease to continue our argument with Reality.

Imagine that you're standing in a mighty river and trying to walk upstream. The river seems to relentlessly

The Natural Way

battle you; it just won't stop pounding you and pushing against you.

Sometimes our lives can feel like that.

But notice that the river has nothing against you; it's just going the way it's going.

It's not the river's job—Existence's job—to get in accord with us; it's vast and we're an atom. Rather, it's our job to get in accord with it—by letting go, by turning around and letting it carry us.

When we're floating down the river, when we've let go of our resistance to it, our sight improves. We're not so preoccupied by the struggle, and we can see things that we couldn't have seen otherwise. We can see opportunities perhaps, or our energy can move in ways that it could not have done before.

But what about giving correction then? Is it ever appropriate? Aren't there times, for instance, when the arithmetic teacher must show her student the mistake he's making in doing fractions?

Yes. But it's worth mentioning a very interesting study that was done concerning teachers and students. What the researchers measured was the ratio of "positive" to "negative" feedback that the teacher was giving to each student and to the class in general. And what they found was this:

The teacher needed to create a positive context for each student before correcting them.

Specifically, teachers had to make at least three-quarters of their comments "positive," telling the student what she was doing right, what was good about her work, and so on. When the teachers did that, the students were very motivated and did well.

However, if the "negative"—corrective—comments to the students increased above one-quarter of all comments the students lost motivation, became apathetic or rebellious, and did poorly.

In any situation, then, we want to be as patient as possible and whenever possible wait until we can push the swing in the direction it's already going, in the "fruitful" or "nurturing" direction. Then we're watering and nurturing the seed of what we do want. We're turning on a light instead of trying to fight the darkness.

Let's take another example, one from Ken Keyes: Suppose the cook's putting too much salt in the soup. So we mention that. Now either the cook is going to say that he didn't realize that and he cuts down the salt, or he defends his "position." In the face of that, it's futile to keep pointing out the "error" to him. Then he would just set his heels in self-righteousness about his position.

The first thing we can do is drop our resistance to the situation. Maybe we eat a little less soup or skip the soup part of the meal. We let go of our attachment that the soup has to be a certain way. We relax and let Reality be the way it is.

The Natural Way

But sooner or later the soup will be a bit less salty, perhaps by accident. Then we naturally respond with our pleasure and appreciation. "You know, I noticed the soup was a little less salty today. It tasted really good. Thank you for that."

And this is not just about salty soup. During the Cuban missile crisis in 1962, President Kennedy received a threatening, bellicose letter from Chairman Khruschev. Then, some hours later, he received a more conciliatory message. No one knew what to do.

It was JFK's brother Bobby who suggested the solution: Ignore the first message; respond to the second.

This approach takes more patience, but it has one great advantage—it works like crazy. And it supports relationships, too, rather than alienating them.

Researchers did a study of couples, and they found that they could predict who would stay together and who would break apart from just one kind of observation: The ratio of positive to negative comments that they said to each other.

The couples that stayed together, on average, said five times as many positive as negative comments to each other. On the other hand, the couples that broke apart, on average, said one-and-a-half times as many negative as positive comments to each other. That one thing could predict the outcome.

What we give attention to expands.

Pt 1—Happiness

What we nourish, with our attention, grows.

Let's now go back to the dragon. What would be the most fundamental way of dealing with it?

Well, suppose we "woke up" and discovered that our fight with the dragon was in a dream? Upon waking up from the dream, the problem would simply dissolve. It would become irrelevant, like our childhood toys left in the closet and no longer used. It's not that anything was "wrong" with our childhood toys; it's just that we move on to other things.

That is about what happens when we let go of our stories about the world, ourselves, and other people, and how it, we, or them are supposed to be better or different in some way.

From that letting-go place, we can then nurture the situation in ways that we couldn't have done before. Then the beautiful, natural seed latent in the situation will tend to evolve even though we're not trying to "improve" anything or anybody anymore.

Then, replacing our desiring of this or that, we're "inspired" to act in some way. Our inner energy moves in some way concerning that situation, perhaps, but without our clinging to some particular outcome, without insisting that it all has to turn out some particular way.

All of this doesn't mean we can't set boundaries if that is appropriate. It does not mean that we always stay in every situation; it doesn't mean that we're necessarily

The Natural Way

passive. Indeed, it's possible that we may even need to be a warrior. The natural actions that will move from our inner heart and energy—behind all the stories—can't be predicted.

But they will tend to produce more harmonious and fruitful results, since we've let go of the compulsion that something or somebody needs to be different. We're able to appreciate this beautiful Reality just as it is, while it evolves in its own organic way.

CHAPTER 4

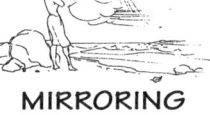
MIRRORING

When we do need to set a boundary of some kind, hopefully we can do so without putting anyone out of our heart. Why? For our own sake. When we're clinging to a story about how something or somebody should have been different in the past or should be different now, our heart hurts.

Check it out for yourself. Look inside and notice that anytime there's a judgment or condemnation about some aspect of Existence, there's a feeling of tightness and disconnection and contraction inside.

Jesus addressed this point. He talked about love a lot, and he talked about what makes unconditional love possible—non-judgmentalness. He talked about this in many ways:

"Judge not that ye be not judged."

"Let he who is without sin cast the first stone."

"Before you judge the speck in your brother's eye, look at the log in your own eye."

This approach is about letting go of our resistance to any part of Reality being the way it is. It's about falling in love with Existence just as it is.

Once again the mind jumps in and says, "But then how will this world ever be 'improved'?" Mysteriously, it's only when we've begun to fall in love with this world, and all aspects of the people and things in it, that we can truly begin to nurture that seed to a more mature state.

The seed doesn't get more perfect, but it does evolve into a more developed form, perhaps a tree or a blade of grass or a rose bush—when we "allow" it to, when we nurture it, when we drop our aversion to any part of Existence and open our heart to all of it instead.

And not coincidentally, we feel much better. We feel connected, whole, joyful.

It's a good test for whatever spiritual or other path we're following in life. If that path is resulting in more open-heartedness, it's probably a fruitful path for us. If it's not, then what's the point?

No matter how many great truths we're learning or how many peak experiences we're having, or how many "undesirable" things or people we're wiping out, is it leading to more love in our heart, more love in the world?

Because the world is just you and I multiplied a few billion times. If it doesn't start in your heart and mine, where will it start? And isn't a more loving world, a world where we can truly love each other, what we really want?

From a place of loving Existence as it is, we're far more able to potentially turn on a light instead of fighting with the darkness, nurturing that seed instead of trying to "improve" it from a place of fear, resentment or anger, which only leads to more of the same.

The world is basically a big mirror for us. What we see and experience "out there" is basically a reflection of what's going on inside us. We see what we're looking for, what we put our attention on.

The resistance we feel inside us to anything in this Existence is mirrored by our external experience. Why? Because it is our stories of the world and the beings in it that determines our experience of the world, and thus our actions in it. Our experience of the world also determines our vibration, and thus what we "magnetize" to us.

When we approach any part of the world from fear or anger—aversion—we're adding to the collective fear and anger in the world. And our actions tend to create more fear and anger and grief in ourselves and others.

Conversely, when we approach the world with love we're adding to the collective love in the world. How else can a world that loves itself come about except through you and me?

The Natural Way

When we let go of our stories about what's "wrong" and about how whoever or whatever "should" be different, we're in a place of vastly greater possibilities.

Do we want the world to change? Let it begin with us then, inside. "As we change, the world changes," James Allen said. Each little bit of open-heartedness that we add inside leads to greater open-heartedness in the world, leads to that seed beginning to grow to its possibility.

That's why Jesus, when asked what was the greatest commandment, said that it was to love God and love our neighbor.

Those two are ultimately the same thing, because if we're not loving our neighbor yet we're not truly loving God either. Because God is our neighbor; God shows up as you and me and our neighbor and our "enemy" and the sky and the flowers in the field.

Imagine a wave on the ocean. Actually, the "wave" only exists within our mind. We look at some part of Existence and define it as something—"This is a wave."

But there's really only the Ocean, now showing up as this wave, now showing up as that wave. It's all just the Ocean, "waving." It's all just One Energy, One Source, showing up as you and me and everybody else and the stars and the mountains and the rivers. And the smiles and tears and the "beautiful" and the "ugly" and the "good" and the "bad"—all of it.

Lao-Tzu pointed out that things spring into existence in our mind as opposites. As soon as we form the concept of "up" we've also formed the concept of "down." "Up" literally has no meaning without the meaning of "down." They come into existence together.

So too with "long" and "short," "hot" and "cold," "day" and "night," "mountains" and "valleys." Can there be a mountain without a valley? No. As soon as a mountain is created, a valley is created at the same time. They go together.

Can we have sun without shadow? No. As soon as we step out into the sun, a shadow is created at the same time. If we want to eliminate all shadows we'd have to eliminate the sun as well. If we wanted to eliminate all "negativities" in Existence, we'd have to eliminate Existence itself.

Paradoxically, when we cease our argument with the "shadows" of Existence, the overall light in ourselves and in the world increases. Then we do whatever we do, but from a different place. We may still work to save the environment, for example, but no longer from a place of fear or clutching or aversion or make-wrong.

Then we're more relaxed, and we do what we do to nurture the garden of this world without clinging to our stories about it and how it's supposed to turn out. And our hearts begin to fill with the unique internal joy that is the hallmark of unaddressed love.

The Natural Way

Jesus emphasized the unaddressed nature of love. He said that if we just love those who love us, well, that's what everybody does. And if we're just good to those who are good to us, again it's not such a big deal because that's what we all do.

He said where our hearts really learn to open is when we can accept the "unacceptable," when we can love the "unlovable." He wanted us to see what the world looked like when we dropped our resistance to it.

He wanted us to see what the world looked like when we saw through all our stories about it.

We can't really know that even a single story is true. Stories are just stories. What exists is just Reality, beneath all the categories and beliefs, just as It is.

When we can love this world just as it is, with all of its horrors and beauties and tragedies and joys, then we're beginning to truly nurture that beautiful seed.

Just as you can't be any different in this moment, nothing else can either. Nothing can help being the way it is. As we begin to see this, we begin to forgive the world—and ourselves and others—for being what it is.

If you were born with the exact same genetic DNA as someone else, and you went through the exact same experiences they did, you'd probably have made the same decisions they did.

If you look back at your life, isn't it true that you've done the best you can? You or somebody else may think that parts of it weren't good enough, but weren't you always doing the best you knew how at that time?

Well everybody else is the same way. Everybody at all times is doing the best they know how to do at that moment. Even when the results are tragic, it was still the best that could be done at the time. If you or I or any other actor in the drama could have been more wise, more conscious, more mature in any given moment, we would have been.

It doesn't mean that we condone all actions. We still may need to set up appropriate boundaries of some kind. As Ken Keyes said, loving someone doesn't necessarily mean that we buy into their act.

What it means is just that we let go of our internal resistance to Reality being that way in that form.

It's almost as if Existence is playing Hide and Seek with us, and saying: "Can you love me like this? Can you love me like that? And what about this part of me?"

As Byron Katie says, how do we know that everything that happens is for the highest good? Because it happens. How do we know that the wind blowing is for the highest good? Because it's blowing.

CHAPTER 5

KINDNESS

There is immense suffering in this world. Even as we read or hear this, there are people in incredible pain in hospitals and elsewhere, there are people feeling lonely and isolated in prisons, there are people being tortured and violated and abused, there are animals suffering in "tight confinement" on factory farms.

Some people are starving, or watching their dreams starve. Some are feeling anxiety or terror or unbearable grief. Some are feeling hopeless or filled with hate. And there are many other forms of suffering in this world.

And there is the suffering in our own hearts. You know, that sense of "disjointedness" inside us that we carefully push down and ignore, but that is there if we really look?

Pt 1—Happiness

This is not a Pollyanna view of life where the unpleasant and the painful are ignored or denied and only the "beautiful" is recognized. There is suffering in this world and in ourselves, along with joy.

The Buddha said that he taught one thing only: "Suffering and the end of suffering."

When we can move from seeing whatever-it-is as "wrong, evil, ugly, unfair" to "suffering and the end of suffering," we stop contributing to the suffering in the world and in ourselves—the suffering brought about by our resistance to some part of Existence.

Part of that resistance is our clinging to various things. We cling to people and places and things gone by. We cling to our beliefs and "truths" hoping they will make us a little more secure in this insecure world.

Our grasping, clutching, manipulating, the quality of insistence about what we want, is also part of our suffering. When we can drop our insistence about getting whatever, then we simply move however our inner energy moves us. And it results in whatever it results in. Existence is free to be more natural, more itself; it's free to begin blossoming to a new state of perfection.

Our ideas of how other people or the world or ourselves should be different is also part of our clinging. But again, no part of Existence can help being what it is. It was brought into Existence being that way, conditioned the way it was conditioned.

The Natural Way

Everything expresses a unique part of Existence, and all of it is somehow necessary. "Night" must exist along with "day." "Winter" must exist with "summer." "Pain" must exist along with "pleasure." "Losing" must exist alongside "winning."

To eliminate all the "downs" and just have the "ups" would eliminate Existence itself, because it can't Exist except as all those dualities. As physicists tell us, when an electron comes into being, an anti-electron or positron always comes into existence at the same time. Dualities exist together.

When we can love it all as it is, our hearts open. Love shows up. God shows up here on earth, in you and in me.

If we want God to appear on earth, It has to show up in you and me. It has no other way to appear. God can only appear in your heart and my heart.

When our heart opens, then the divine shows up on earth. Because then we become a channel for divine love, which doesn't discriminate.

As Jesus points out, Existence sends its sun and its rain to saint and sinner alike. It doesn't ask who you are before it sends its warming sun to you. It doesn't ask who you are before it sends its healing rain to you.

And when the rain isn't healing, that's also part of Its healing rain. And when it's night and there's no light, that's also part of Its healing light. And when it's winter and cold, that's also part of Its healing warmth.

We can partake of that divine love when we are willing to love Existence as it is, just as it is, in all its multi-colored hues.

Then we let go of our grasping and clinging and aversion and judgments. Then joy enters our heart.

The Buddha gave us some advice to counteract the suffering of our wanting and clinging and clutching (and the opposite side of the same coin, our aversions). To put it in modern language, he advised reversing the direction of that flow 180 degrees.

He advised cultivating generosity. Generosity in our heart—love. And also generosity in an external sense, giving to the world however we can.

And he advised cultivating this, growing it just like a garden. He knew well that hearts don't grow overnight, but patiently, day by day, when an intention to nurture them exists.

When we're generous, we reverse the suffering of wanting and clinging. We're asking what we can give to this world rather than what we can take from it. We ask how we can nurture this person or this situation and help them or it to blossom rather than manipulating them or it to be different.

We partake of the joy of giving, then. As Francis of Assisi said, "Let me console rather than be consoled...for it is in giving that we receive."

When we can love this world and each other just as it and we are, in all our perfect imperfection, that is our greatest gift.

Where this greatest gift really shows up is in our everyday life. It shows up in how kindly we treat ourselves and each other and the world in our ordinary, day-to-day actions and encounters.

The Dalai Lama, when asked what his religion was, said: "My religion is kindness."

Is our spiritual path showing up as more everyday kindness, more open-heartedness and generosity in our ordinary life? Do we feel more in love with this world, with Existence?

Jesus was a person who loved Existence just as it was, and he wanted us to get a glimpse of what it was that he was seeing.

"Love one another as I have loved you," Jesus said to us.

And he gave us the Golden Rule, which can also be found in the Old Testament and in many other places and sources:

"Treat others in the way that you yourself would want to be treated."

When we can do that, or begin to, we begin to let go of this self-centered little clod of selfish interests and become a channel for something much vaster, not less than Everything.

Then we surrender our little life and our hidden-away misery and unhappiness and grasping and wanting and struggling, and let the energy of Existence move through us in whatever way It wants to.

We follow that inner energy, that inner guidance—which moves by itself and feels like love and possibility rather than fear—and find ourselves doing whatever it is we do without knowing why. There's no rhyme or reason anymore, it's all just happening by itself.

Notice your breathing. It was happening before you noticed it just now and it will keep on happening when your attention has moved elsewhere.

It's happening by itself, along with the digestion of your food and the circulation of your blood and the balancing of your hormones and the firing of neurons in your brain and literally countless other things.

So too, all of Existence is happening by itself. When we let go of all our judgments, we begin to cooperate with it, to dance with it. We begin to meet it just in the moment, without pre-conditions or stories. We begin to love it as it is.

Then we're turning on a light instead of fighting with darkness or the furniture. Then we're waking up from our waking dream of stories about Reality, and we find that our problems either disappear or that we can approach them in a more fruitful way.

Reversing the flow.

The Natural Way

Gratitude also reverses the flow of clinging. Instead of complaining about whatever, we tune into the perfect imperfection of Existence, including ourselves, and we begin to take joy in it. We let go.

We begin to tune into the incredible beauty of it all, including the waves and violets and even all the "wrong" things we see.

All of it is necessary, ceaselessly weaving back and forth between day and night, winter and summer, sunshine and rain, health and disease, youth and old age, winning and losing, pleasure and pain, joy and sorrow, life and death, darkness and light.

CHAPTER 6

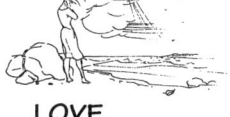

LOVE

The greatest achievement, in my opinion, is not to be some superhuman person who never feels the ordinary human feelings of grief or fear or pain. All of that is just as much a part of life as joy, excitement and pleasure.

Our impulses are almost constantly tugging at us. "Do this," they say. "Do that." Cajoling us through our desires and judgments and aversions and so on.

But we can just watch all that. That's what the Buddha and many other people pointed out. We can just watch those impulses and stories and let them be there.

We can let them appear on their own and disappear on their own without buying into them, without picking them up. We can accept that they're there without acting on them.

The Natural Way

We can watch them, just like watching leaves floating down a stream, or clouds floating across the sky, or waves rising and falling. They rise and fall by themselves if we just watch them without identifying with them.

Deep, silent stillness helps a lot with this. "Silence is the greatest teacher," Ramana Maharshi said.

Just going into a period of sitting in silence every day, and watching the parade of desires and intentions and resentments and stories and beliefs surface again and again in our mind helps us to see that they're just productions and projections of the mind.

This quality of bare witnessing of our internal stream of thoughts and feelings, using the same love and acceptance that we can bring to the outside world, has been called vipassana, mindfulness, natural attention and many other things.

Basically it means being aware of our thoughts and feelings as just thoughts and feelings. It means accepting them and watching them but giving them no energy, not getting involved. The alternative is to identify with the thoughts and go off on a "train of thought." That's our living, waking daydream of being fast asleep.

When we can just watch that whole internal parade, with great love and acceptance but without identifying with it, we have more equanimity about it all. We're more willing to let things flow into and out of our life, to love this life as it is.

Pt 1—Happiness

We know that everything will change and that everything and everybody that appears in our life will disappear someday, that whatever is born will die, that whatever or whoever feels pleasure will also have to feel pain. And we can make our peace with all of that.

We can surrender, as Mohammed, Rumi, Hafez, Rabiya and other mystic and poetic Muslims and Sufis have recommended.

To what? To the Beloved, to Existence itself, from which we have never ever been separate. So in a sense we surrender to ourselves, to Life. We surrender to the great and majestic Mystery that we can't really understand.

Is this process done all at once? No more than a farmer can plant seeds and harvest all at once. It takes time and patience. And of course we'll have many "setbacks," times when we can't be as conscious or as loving as at other times. That's all part of the process too.

If we meet in the supermarket tomorrow, will you necessarily find me loving and kind and conscious? Not necessarily. Maybe I'm having a bad day. Maybe I didn't sleep last night. Maybe I'm caught up in some drama or story in that moment and I'm not as awake or kind to you as I would wish to be when I'm more relaxed.

Your journey is the same in that respect. There will be times when you're caught in some way, when you're identifying with the belief or story and you're contracted inside. It's all just part of it.

The Natural Way

When we do contract inside, we can say "yes" to that too; we can say "yes to the no."

When we contract, and we will many times, we can love that contraction too, and just keep coming back to our intention to nurture our heart and the garden of this world as best we can.

We can just water that seed each day and it will sprout and blossom in its own natural time.

From one point of view we're just molecules and atoms and quarks ceaselessly vibrating and interweaving and sometimes spraying up as a "Mary" or a "Bill" or a "willow tree" or a "daisy" for a little while.

From another point of view, if we pull back to the viewpoint of the immensely vast stretch of galaxies, we're not even as noticeable as a grain of sand on the beach.

And here we are in between for a little while.

And during that little while, love is all that really matters. Isn't it true? When we're lying on our deathbed, as dying people report, we mainly remember the times others loved us and the times we loved them.

CHAPTER 7

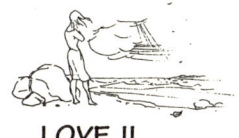

LOVE II

Love is all that really matters.

Not just love for our loved ones, those who treat us well, but love for everything that's left over too, as Jesus said. Even love for our "enemies" in this drama. Yes to everything in this beautiful, mysterious Existence.

Love that's not conditional on something or someone being some way, that's not addressed to somewhere in particular, that doesn't leave any being or thing out.

Then our greatest achievement as humans is just to live an ordinary life. To love and laugh and cry and weep bitter tears at times, and wash the dishes and take care of each other.

To water the garden and prepare the meals and deal with the problems and raise our children as best we can and love the whole process of it all, knowing that we'll make many "mistakes."

Knowing that this little spray that the ocean has thrown up is perfectly imperfect in its ordinariness and humanness, and that that is its greatness.

To accept our humanity is to accept that we're all saint and sinner, we all have the potential of Hitler and Mother Teresa inside.

So we study the process we're going through on the way to some ideal, because we know that the process is the real product. We know that the means we use to achieve some great end is the real end we achieve.

Accepting our humanity means accepting that we're capable of being insensitive and cruel at one moment and kind and compassionate at another, intelligent and wise at one time and ignorant and foolish at another. As humans we embody many contradictions, just as all beings do and as Existence itself does.

When we can accept and love those contradictions in ourselves and others and the world, and just keep patiently nurturing our love of Existence, pointing out what's beautiful and true in each person, how magnificent they are in their ordinary beingness, then the divine is coming through us and once again showing up on earth. In your heart. In my heart.

Then the Ocean is expressing its Heart through your wave or my wave. But really there is no "your wave" or "my wave." It's all just the Ocean doing it. It's the Ocean that's doing everything whatsoever.

And we can trust That, without feeling that it needs to look some particular way or to reach some particular outcome. We can trust it knowing that the black clouds are as necessary as the white clouds, knowing that sadness is as necessary as joy and has its own beauty.

We can trust the same Existence that's beating our heart to take care of everything else too, in a way that we can't really understand with our mind but we can feel with our heart.

So we do what we do. We play our part as impeccably and kindly as we can, knowing all the while that it's a great privilege to be here, to be able to appreciate this Existence, to allow the Existence to appreciate Itself, so to speak, through us.

We nurture as best we can that seed in our heart, accepting our ordinary, magnificent and contradictory humanity along the way.

We nurture as best we can this seed that we call the world, accepting the magnificence of its ordinariness. A flower. A leaf. A pair of eyes. A heart. Yes, even our own ceaseless judgments about what's "good" and "bad."

Then that seed of love begins to grow into its natural potential, to evolve to the flower that lies within it. But there's no hurry. Everything takes its own time, like a field of flowers growing.

The Natural Way

And we can cooperate with the vast blossoming of Existence by appreciating the way it is now, by allowing ourselves to see the perfection of that seed as it is now, and nurturing it as best we can. We do our best to turn on a light instead of cursing the darkness. Then things can evolve to whatever's next.

Lao-Tzu, the founder of Taoism, said:

"Rejoice in the way things are."

I love that. Notice that he didn't say to grudgingly put up with the way things are. No; he said:

"*Rejoice* in the way things are."

Rejoice in this world just as it is.

Rejoice in others just the way they are.

Rejoice in yourself just the way you are.

Rejoice in your life just the way it is.

Then you feel the blessing, whenever you do, of an opening heart. You feel the growing joy of appreciating Existence in all the forms it presents. You feel more and more in love with this beautiful Existence, which comes alive within your heart and the hearts of others.

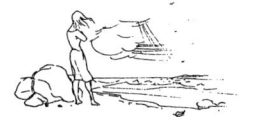

PART 2
Vitality

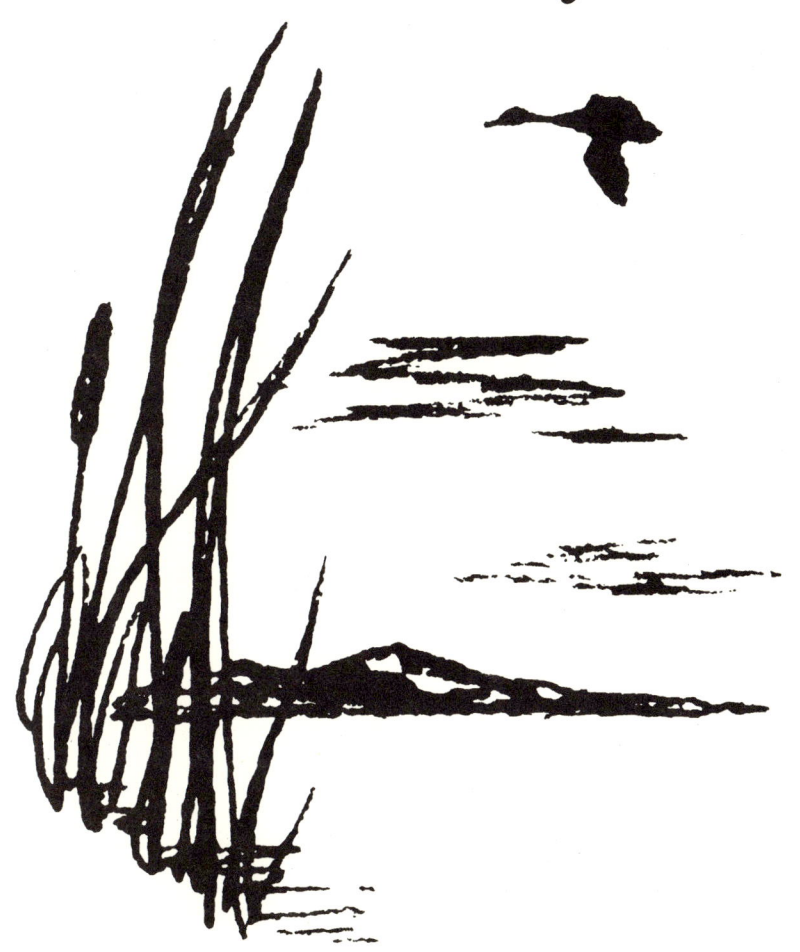

CHAPTER 8

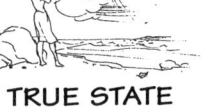

TRUE STATE

We've been talking about the warm Intelligence in the world at large and also within ourselves, and how that can be trusted. Now let's see how this perspective might apply in a very practical area—the body.

Seeing how it works at the physical level can shed a lot of light on the general principle of the natural way of things. So how might this perspective of trusting the natural Intelligence work in the dimension of health and disease?

First, we should note that it is possible to be happy even if the body is badly impaired. Ramana Maharshi, dying in extreme pain from cancer, proved that. Many other spiritual teachers have proven that also. But it takes more consciousness.

The Natural Way

Conversely, if the body is enjoying its inherent and natural vitality and lightness it can be quite helpful to our consciousness. So let's explore this area.

We can begin our exploration by looking at the real state of our body. If we want to know the true present state of our body, it's quite easy to find out. All we have to do is go without eating for a couple of days, taking in water and nothing else for a little while.

There are people, even professional people, who will tell us that this will kill us, that it can be dangerous and so forth. And in one way that statement is right and in another way it's not right. You see, it all depends on how toxic we are.

If our body is very toxic, as many of our bodies are, we're in for a bit of a shock. What we do at the end of the two days is stand in front of a mirror and just take a mental snapshot of how we look and feel. What most of us are going to find is that we don't look and feel so hot. We're feeling and seeing the true state of our body now, and it can be a bit alarming.

For most of us, our tongue will be coated. This is reflecting the actual state of the intestinal system of most of us—coated with stuff. The eyes might look dull or bloodshot or they might burn or feel uncomfortable in some way. The skin most likely won't look so great, and can be anywhere from itchy to blotchy. Or we may look bloated. Other signs can occur.

We may feel rather fatigued, low-energy, lethargic. We may feel sick. It's quite possible we'll develop signs of a cold or flu. Allergies may appear or get worse, or we might have a bad headache. All these things and more are signs of a toxic body.

It's good to be careful and intelligent about fasting for a little while, precisely because some of us are so toxic, often without knowing it.

For most of us, the symptoms will be a variation of the above. But some of us are more toxic still, and the two-day fast will reveal that. So we may not want to do it except under the supervision of a professional. Only we can say; we're responsible for ourselves. Incidentally, if a professional is used they should be *trained in fasting*.

The above is particularly true if we're taking any prescription drugs or have a clinical illness. We have to trust our intuition and intelligence here. But let's err on the side of caution and safety.

In fact, the first time I fasted I had to stop my fast in the middle of the third day because I was so ill. I had a fever, I was stuffed up, had a runny nose, was very weak and ached all over and felt absolutely miserable.

What was going on? My body's toxicity had been concealed from me and now it was being revealed. My body was starting to unload its toxic burden, and it was not feeling like fun. My feeling so ill was an indication of how toxic I truly was.

The Natural Way

You may need to stop after a single day or even a few hours; you be the judge of what's right for you. But I'll tell you, it's an interesting experiment to conduct if it's feasible, because it's such an eye-opener.

By the way, what do you think happens if your body is really detoxed and you fast for a couple of days?

The answer is: nothing.

Yes, that's right—nothing. When our body is truly cleansed inside and we don't eat, nothing happens. We feel just the same as before—that is, energetic, vital and with a great sense of well-being.

If our body is cleansed inside and we fast for 48 hours and then look in the mirror, our eyes will look bright and shiny, our tongue will be pink, our skin will glow with health and we'll feel great—just as before. Indeed, a cleansed body can fast for weeks and feel fine the whole time. This is our natural state.

And it makes sense. When we lived in the wild, our food supply was capable of being interrupted at any time for various reasons. Our body had to be capable of easily handling periodic interruptions in food supply—and even of benefiting from them.

CHAPTER 9

TOXIFICATION

The general concept of health in our society and other industrialized ones is that health is an absence of symptoms. I know this paradigm well, having lived with it for many years.

The general feeling for me was feeling "okay" but easily tired or fatigued, not really having a whole lot of energy. I'd get bad headaches sometimes, or unexplained aches somewhere. I got frequent "colds" and "flus." I had asthma sometimes, and allergies to one thing or another all the time. All this I considered just a normal state of affairs; that's how you were supposed to feel.

I'd grown up on a more-or-less average American diet. On an average morning we might have bacon and eggs with white toast and pasteurized juice. For lunch perhaps a bologna or peanut butter sandwich or a BLT. For dinner perhaps steak or meat loaf or lamb chops or fish, with a couple of over-cooked vegetables and, for dessert, perhaps some canned peaches in sugar syrup. I drank lots of milk and sugary colas.

In fact, this was considered a good diet, not just by my family but by everyone we knew. My family, to the best of its ability, was putting the best food on the table that it knew of. We considered it a good diet.

Once a year or so I'd get a physical, at school or elsewhere. I was always pronounced in excellent health. Yet I had this nagging feeling, deep down, that all wasn't quite right. I couldn't put my finger on it, though.

I wished I had more energy, but people do get tired sometimes. I wished I didn't get so many colds and flus, but of course the "Asian flu" this year was particularly nasty, and so what did I expect? Headaches were normal —everybody got them now and then. And so on.

When I was 21 a friend handed me, by great good fortune, a copy of Adelle Davis' book *Let's Eat Right To Keep Fit.* Suddenly the light dawned. That's what it felt like, because for the first time I made the connection that my diet actually had something to do with my health and physical well-being. What a concept!

What I really respect about Adelle Davis is that she was doing her utmost to be helpful, given the knowledge that she had available to her.

Pt 2—Vitality

    She made the point that I should eat whole-grain foods instead of white, devitalized breads, pastas, rices. She discussed Hans Seyle's research which showed that all stresses of any kind induced bodily responses which, continued over time, added to the body's toxicity. She made me see the importance of getting enough vitamins and minerals in my diet, and since stresses were so high in modern life, that it was good to make sure by using vitamin and mineral supplements. I should also, she said, make sure I was getting enough protein and fat and enough (pasteurized) milk.

    This was a big step forward for me. My paradigm previously had been basic helplessness about my health, that health or lack of it was something—like the flu or a headache—that just happened to you. A good part of this paradigm was a dependence upon professionals.

    Basically, I considered that my health was something I got from seeing the right professionals and getting the right drugs or procedures whenever something went wrong with my body.

    If I had a headache I needed aspirin. If I had high cholesterol I needed anti-cholesterol medication. If my tonsils became inflamed I needed someone to cut them out for me. My health was dependent upon externals—access to the right drugs, treatments, etc.

    The new paradigm from Adelle Davis was a great shift because I saw that my health depended, much more than I'd previously thought, upon my own choices each day, particularly in the area of diet.

If I ate whole-wheat bread I got more vitamin B and E and minerals than if I ate the white bread. If I got enough vitamin C every day, infections would clear up quicker. Getting enough protein would tend to keep my liver healthy; taking supplements of vitamin A would tend to keep my eyes healthy. These were things that I had some control over.

Notice, though, that this perspective is still one of *externality*. Now, instead of needing the right procedures, drugs, etc., I needed the right vitamins and minerals and special health foods and so on. Health was still basically dependent upon special stuff from the outside.

Later on, I migrated to a variation of this external paradigm. Now health was dependent upon getting the right herbs, essences, alternative treatments, energetic enhancers, etc. If I had a cold I needed echinacea, if I was depressed I needed St. John's wort; if I wasn't feeling so good it was because I hadn't gotten a spinal adjustment lately or used my homeopathic preparation.

In fact, each new paradigm was a step forward, and I had great success in clearing up various conditions in both myself and others by advice on various supplements —and also what to avoid.

I began to realize the importance of the latter. For instance, I learned that it was good to avoid jellies and jams and sugar sodas and white-flour breads and other products if I didn't want to feel fatigued a lot.

Why? Because refined sugar and starch products were "empty calories"—deficient in all sorts of vitamins, for instance, causing the body to use more of its own meager store of vitamins to digest them. That in turn creates over time a deficiency of certain vitamins that are intimately involved in the production of energy.

This made sense and it worked. I found that when I ate whole-grain cereal, pasta, breads, etc. and avoided refined sugar and starch in its various forms I really did have more energy. My blood sugar, instead of going up and down like a roller-coaster, tended to stabilize.

A candy bar would give me "quick energy"—lots of sugar right away. But the rapid rise in sugar would cause my pancreas to overreact and secrete too much insulin, which then drove my blood sugar *down* and caused me to feel blue, irritable or low-energy. When I ate brown rice or pasta instead, the complex starch was digested slowly, releasing a steady supply of glucose into the bloodstream for hours. My energy became more steady.

As another example, I learned to avoid deep-fried foods and fried foods in general such as french fries and donuts and fried chicken. Why? Because fats go into cell walls, and heated oils form toxic chemicals that damage the structure of cells, making them more susceptible to such things as cancer or infectious agents.

The Natural Way

From Nathan Pritikin's work I learned that fats in general were harmful in high quantities. He pointed out that the body dealt with fat not in terms of weight but in terms of calories.

So I learned that whole milk, 3% fat by weight, was 49% fat when measured by calories. Eggs were 70% fat, a steak or pork chop was 70% fat, a turkey leg was 35% fat, most fish were 40% to 70% fat, etc. These were all high-fat foods. By contrast, most fruits and vegetables were around 5% fat and most grains around 10%—much, much lower.

I found out that the average diet of industrialized societies was around 40% fat by calories and the average diet of the Hunzas—considered the healthiest people on earth—was around 7%. Quite a difference.

I learned that my high-fat diet tended to lay down deposits in my arteries leading to high-blood pressure and strokes and heart disease. My high-fat diet was also correlated in various studies to a much greater incidence of degenerative diseases such as cancer, diabetes, stroke, arthritis, multiple sclerosis, etc.

These were the new paradigms I learned and they were very helpful. But there were more valuable ones to come.

CHAPTER 10

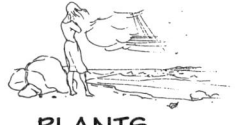

PLANTS

An important step occurred early in 1990 when I became a true vegetarian. I'd been flirting with the idea for some years, but hadn't really crossed over. Then I read a book by John Robbins called *Diet For A New America*. Once again, the light dawned.

That book made three main assertions about being a vegetarian:
 1. It's much better for your personal health.
 2. It relieves animals of all kinds of suffering.
 3. It's much better for the environment.

What's great about Robbins is that he didn't just make these assertions, but patiently gathered together all of the evidence to definitively prove them.

I had known for some time that being a vegetarian

was better for my personal health. There is actually a large body of research now showing that vegetarians live longer, have fewer diseases, have more endurance and so on. (See John Robbins' book or *Handbook for Humans* by this author for more detail about this.)

This knowledge was enough to make me a partial vegetarian, but only a partial one. I liked the taste of meat and fish and poultry too much to ever give them up completely, I thought.

Also in Robbins' book is a very clear demonstration of the relative costs to the environment of meat-eating versus plant-eating. And what it boils down to is this: That feeding plants to animals and then harvesting the animals for food is very inefficient—it uses many more natural resources, and results in much greater pollution, than eating the plants directly.

For example, it takes 20 times as much land to feed a meat-eater as to feed a vegetarian. It takes 100 times as much water to produce a pound of meat as it does to grow a pound of grain. It takes 20 times as much fossil fuel to support a meat-eater, and vastly greater amounts of sewage and toxins are produced in the process. And so on; many more examples could be given.

That was powerful, but it still didn't convince me to become a complete vegetarian. What did it was reading about the animals and what was happening to them.

To put it succinctly, the way livestock increasingly

are raised in modern societies is inhuman and torturous. Livestock animals are thought of as economic units which can be crammed into gigantic warehouses where extreme over-crowding is the norm and where they often never see the light of day in their entire lives.

Many livestock animals are kept in such a way that they can scarcely move their entire lives. Imagine what your life would feel like if you had to spend all of it in the space of a closet. And there's many more details.

Then I realized that I was responsible for this, since every time I ate a piece of meat I was helping to create the demand that supported this system. And I gave up meat that very day.

But here's an interesting note: I thought that giving up meat and fish completely would be difficult, and it was, more or less—for about four months. At the end of that time I noticed with fascination that I simply didn't desire meat anymore. The desire just wasn't there. Not only that, but I actually preferred vegetables and fruits and whole grains. This was a revelation to me.

Now let's examine the first item, that vegetarianism is better for our personal health. And since the research has already been mentioned, let's examine it in a more common-sense way, by observing the structure of various animal bodies including ours. What do we find?

A very notable feature of carnivores—designed by nature as meat-eaters—is their intestinal system, which is about three times the length of their trunk. Relatively speaking, this is a very short length. Why so short?

Have you ever left a piece of meat sitting out on a counter for a few days? The meat starts turning black and putrid, filled with a witches' brew of toxic chemicals and micro-organisms. The carnivore's system wants to get rid of meat before it putrefies and becomes poisonous. Its short intestinal system is designed for the rapid digestion and expulsion of meat before that happens.

In contrast, our intestinal system, like that of the *herbivores* (plant-eating animals) is about 12 times the length of our trunk. It's designed for the relatively long times required for the digestion of plants.

When we eat a piece of meat, it stays in our body much longer than it stays in the body of a carnivore. During that time, the meat does indeed putrefy, releasing toxic poisons that are absorbed into our system, resulting in *autotoxemia*. We'll return to that later.

The digestion of meat (or any other animal protein, such as eggs) results in the release of a powerful systemic poison, uric acid, in large quantities. The carnivore's body is perfectly equipped to handle this. Its liver produces an enzyme, uricase, which can neutralize large quantities of uric acid. In contrast, the bodies of humans and other herbivores *do not produce uricase at all.*

Let's look at our teeth and hands. A carnivore has sharp, pointed teeth and sharp claws, designed for the ripping and tearing of flesh and the rapid killing of prey. In contrast, we have hands perfectly designed for the plucking of fruit from trees and the gathering of vegetables from the land. And our teeth are designed for the crushing and grinding of fibrous plant foods.

A carnivore's stomach secretes about 10 times more hydrochloric acid than ours. That is why a dog can eat a piece of meat off the floor and not worry about bacteria. A carnivore has an acid saliva and acid urine. We have an alkaline saliva and urine, like all herbivores.

The list could go on. For example, carnivores have no problem with cholesterol. They produce an enzyme, cholinesterase, that can neutralize an almost unlimited amount of cholesterol. That is why my cat can eat fatty meat all day and never get heart disease. In contrast, our bodies have a hard time with ingested cholesterol.

And think of the psychological aspect. If you're out walking and you come across an animal hit by a car and dying by the side of the road, do you salivate and think of lunch? Probably not. If anything, we feel sadness.

If we were true carnivores, our mouth would water at the delicious prospect of eating that animal right there and licking its blood. Instead, if we're talking about foods as they're created by nature, we're attracted to things like an orange or a ripe banana.

CHAPTER 11

PLANTS II

It's enlightening, too, to look at the differing effects which animal and plant foods have on the body.

For instance, meats—and animal foods in general—have no fiber in them. Why is this notable? Because the fiber in plant foods absorbs water. This keeps the *bolus* or food mass moving along in the intestines.

But a bolus of meat, containing no fiber to retain water, becomes dry as it progresses through the intestine. Thus its progress slows down and becomes somewhat difficult, which can lead to constipation, gas, irritation, inflammation and the absorption of toxins.

Animal foods also contain much higher amounts of sodium. Our bodies evolved over a hundred million years of tree living to conserve sodium and excrete potassium.

Why? Because our plant-based diet contained a lot of potassium and not much sodium.

Yet the diets of industrialized societies have huge amounts of sodium (animal foods, added salt, soy sauce, etc.) and not much potassium (natural plant foods). Our potassium-to-sodium intake ratio is only about 0.4-to-1 now, compared to our original ratio of over 40-to-1.

Well, so what?

Consider this. It's a simplification, but not overly so, to say that the bloodstream contains sodium and the cells contain potassium. These two molecules compete for water. When the body contains too much sodium and not enough potassium, water is drawn out of the cells.

When this dehydration happens to the cells in the brain, the resulting severe headache is indistinguishable from what's known as a "migraine." Indeed, everyone I've ever come across who had "migraine headaches" found that they could completely eliminate them by drastically lowering the salt in their diet to a natural level.

To do so it helps very much to take up a vegetarian diet, since fruits and vegetables tend to be low in sodium and high in potassium. And it's also useful to identify sources of salt such as soy sauce and animal foods and virtually all processed or restaurant foods. In doing so, the result is a much lower incidence of such diseases as stroke, high blood pressure, kidney disorders, migraine headaches, etc.

The Natural Way

Finally, we come to the empirical perspective. This very sensibly asks: Who the healthiest peoples on earth? And what do *they* eat?

As it turns out, the healthiest, longest-lived peoples on the planet are generally considered to be the Hunzas of Kashmir in northern Pakistan and the Vilcabambans of Ecuador.

Strikingly, these widely separated peoples have very similar diets. They're both 99-100% vegetarian. They eat organic fresh fruits, vegetables and whole grains, and eat them in a simple, unprocessed form. There's no magic, no secrets. They just eat a fresh, unrefined vegetarian diet and, equally important, avoid almost everything else.

Sir Robert McCarrison wanted to find out if the Hunzas' great health and longevity—they had virtually no degenerative diseases—was the result of diet or something else. So he devised a famous experiment:

He chose white rats because, like humans, they'll eat almost anything. And he divided them into groups. Then he fed the rats different national diets. That is, he fed one group an average British diet, another group an average Indian diet, another group an average Hunza diet and so forth. Then, at an equivalent age of 50 years in a human, he autopsied them.

What he found was remarkable. Each group of rats had developed the diseases characteristic of that human population. The "British" rats, for instance, had diseases

Pt 2—Vitality

characteristic of the British human population, like heart disease and stroke and cancer and diabetes. Similarly, the "Indian" rats developed Indian diseases, and so on.

But what of the "Hunza" rats?

The "Hunza" rats, it seems, developed no diseases. No pathology at all could be found. This is a strong clue that it's the diet of the Hunzas, rather than other factors, that is the determining factor in their health.

The problem isn't just that animal foods tend to contain a lot of fat and toxins and no fiber. The China Project, headed by T. Colin Campbell, studied the link between the diets of 65,000 people and their diseases.

The first finding to come out was that degenerative diseases increased in proportion to dietary fat. But that was not a surprise. What did surprise the researchers was the even higher correlation between those degenerative diseases and the intake of *animal protein*. Or conversely, that a plant-based diet was extremely protective against these same degenerative diseases.

According to anthropologists, the hunter-gatherer phase of human history, about the last million and a half years or so, was always much more "gatherer" than it was "hunter." Until the last 200 years or so, we always ate far more plant foods than animal foods.

The affluence released by the Industrial Revolution changed all that. For the first time in human history it became possible to have meat or other animal food at every meal. From the evidence, the results have been disastrous, as shown by the startling rise in degenerative diseases in the last two centuries.

But can a vegetarian diet offer enough protein?

In modern industrialized societies, we seem to have a cult of protein. This got started from experiments early in the century that showed that animals fed high-protein diets grew faster. Much later it was discovered that the animals also died much sooner, but by then the worship of protein was well on its way.

The average American gets almost 150 grams of protein a day, mostly from animal foods. Yet studies of nitrogen loss show that we only need to replace about 22 grams of protein per day on average. The World Health Organization recommends about 25-35 grams per day. The excess that we get is a stress to the body.

For example, the metabolism of protein generates a lot of acidic toxins, which enter the bloodstream. When concentrated protein is consumed, as in animal foods, the acidic residues have to be neutralized by the body since the bloodstream must be kept alkaline at all cost.

To accomplish this, the body pulls minute amounts of calcium from the bones in order to neutralize the excess acidity in the blood. The amount of calcium that's withdrawn is very small, but continued over decades it results in the bones becoming much more porous—the osteoporosis so prevalent in the elderly today.

It needn't be this way. African Bantu women get far less calcium than American women, only about 400 mg a day, yet birth and suckle an average of nine children without getting osteoporosis. How? Because their diet of mostly fruits, vegetables and grains, like that of the Hunzas, is low in protein.

In fact, researchers discovered that women could not be gotten out of negative calcium balance by even high amounts of calcium supplementation. That result could be achieved, they found, only by lowering the amount of protein in the diet.

What about milk and dairy products, which are so strongly touted for their calcium content? Ironically, the protein in dairy products, creating acidic end-products in the body, more than offsets the calcium provided. The result is a net *loss* of bone calcium over the years. In fact, the countries with the highest dairy consumption have, as well, the highest rates of osteoporosis.

Milk is not a health food on other counts. It has no more fiber than any other animal food. It has long been known as a mucous-producing and clogging food. And I've known a number of people who eliminated bursitis simply by giving up dairy products.

Actually, we're the only animal who consumes dairy products after weaning (not including pets, who must eat what we give them). Can you imagine going up to a cow, getting under it and sucking on its teats? Does that

The Natural Way

appeal to you? It's not something that we'd do in nature. But that's what we're doing in effect when we consume dairy foods.

A low-fat, low-protein diet based on plant foods is sometimes called a *starch-centered diet*. John McDougall, among others, has popularized this kind of diet in his excellent book *The McDougall Program*.

What does such a diet consist of? In essence, meat or other animal food is replaced as the centerpiece of the meal by a starch—such as bread, pasta, cereal, potatoes, yams, rice, etc. The meal is completed by adding fruits or vegetables.

So breakfast on such a diet might be, say, oatmeal with blueberries. Lunch might be a veggie-burger with tomatoes and sprouts on a whole-wheat bun. Dinner might be a vegetable pizza without cheese, or brown rice with grilled vegetables and a salad.

There are many variations and a number of good cookbooks are now available using this diet. It's a good, solid diet that will usually provide sustained energy and a life normally free of various degenerative diseases.

A low-fat, low-protein, plant-based diet is indeed a compelling one for good health.

But an even more powerful paradigm awaited me.

CHAPTER 12

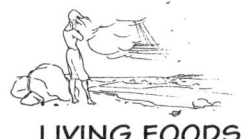

LIVING FOODS

A low-fat, plant-based, starch-centered diet will do wonders for how we feel. In all probability we'll feel more balanced, get fewer or no colds or flus, have more energy and have it more steadily. We'll be likely to live longer and enjoy it more because we'll be much less likely to develop the modern degenerative diseases.

Such a diet has much to recommend it.

But if we really want to feel outrageous energy, if we'd like to feel our body in a whole new way, if we want to feel our body aligned with itself in a way we may not have thought possible—then try raw foods.

Another name for them is *living foods*.

These foods are called "living foods" because the enzymes are still active in them. Above 105°F enzymes

The Natural Way

become damaged and above 129°F all enzymes are just destroyed.

Why does that matter?

Virtually everything that goes on in our bodies does so because of enzymes. Our body makes about 100,000 different kinds of proteins every day to function. Both the making and the functioning of those proteins is possible only with enzymes. From digestion to energy production, from nerve impulses to fighting infections—it's all done with enzymes.

Digestion in particular requires large amounts of enzymes. Raw, living foods come into the body carrying their own enzymes, which contribute to the digestion of these foods. This being so, the body itself has to produce fewer digestive enzymes—which then frees it to allocate its resources to other areas, such as producing energy or detoxifying itself.

The body is marvelous beyond all imagining, but it does not have unlimited resources. At any given time it has a certain amount of resources, which may be termed its *life energy* or *vital energy*. Like a general or CEO, it must allocate its resources among competing demands. If it allocates a lot of resources over here, fewer may be available over there.

Because fresh, raw, living foods need less energy to digest, large amounts of energy and resources are made available for other needs in the body.

Also, the essential nutrients in living foods—the proteins, fats, carbohydrates, vitamins, etc.—come into the body undamaged. That is, the body has undamaged amino acids, fatty acids and so on with which to build and rebuild itself. This also results in greater efficiency in all systems of the body.

So the first thing we'll notice from eating raw foods is a *tremendous* increase in energy. It's the kind of energy we had as a child, a spirited energy that tends to overflow into taking delight in life and feeling connected with it. Because of this, a living food diet often contributes a new dimension to our spiritual journey.

Why this increase in energy? Because a living foods diet closely replicates the diet that we ate in nature, the diet that our bodies evolved and adapted to over tens of millions of years.

Anthropologists say that our predecessors started out as tree shrews about the size of a squirrel, roughly 100 million years ago. We lived in the trees and ate what was available there, namely fruits, nuts and greens. As we grew larger and more like today's primates over time, we continued to be *arboreans*—tree-dwellers—until just a few million years ago.

Thus our body had vast eons of time to perfectly adapt to this living plant-based food kind of diet. Of course, this diet was naturally fresh and uncooked. It was naturally unrefined, organic, high in fiber and vitamins

The Natural Way

and phyto-nutrients. And it was naturally low in fat, salt, toxins and animal protein.

On May 15, 1979 an article appeared in the New York Times describing the work of Alan Walker of Johns Hopkins. With the immense magnification of a scanning electron microscope, Walker found that all kinds of food left minute but characteristic abrasions on teeth, and that by identifying those abrasions he could pinpoint what kind of food an animal had eaten during its lifetime.

Then he applied this technique to the teeth of the various proto-human fossils available, ranging all the way back to 12 million years ago. Here's what he found:

His research found that all of the human ancestors, without exception, were *fruitarians*—living primarily on fruits, with added nuts and greens—until approximately 1.5 million years ago. This means that the body had at least 10.5 million years—and most likely 100 million—to optimize around a fruitarian diet.

Is it any wonder then that the body responds so dramatically to a diet of living plant-based foods? Once again, on that kind of diet, it's getting the kind of raw food that it optimized for over so many millions of years. The result is electric.

But what's the difference, we might ask, between eating a piece of fruit and having a sugared soda? Fruit does have sugar, it's true, but it occurs naturally. This fruit sugar is surrounded by natural fiber and minerals and enzymes, all of which seems to make a great difference in how the body responds to it.

This response isn't just more energy. On a living-food diet there is also an increasing sense of harmony in the body, like a finely-tuned engine, though this comes through most clearly after the body has detoxified.

About 1.5 million years ago we became *omnivores*, eaters of anything, but research shows that even then we received 3 to 4 times as many calories from plants as from animals. This remained true until the advent of the Industrial Revolution a couple of centuries ago.

And as far as cooking goes, researchers believe that we probably began cooking our food in a systematic way only about 15,000-25,000 years ago.

Think about it: The body had 100 million years to adapt to a raw enzyme-rich plant diet, and about 15,000-25,000 years to adapt to a cooked diet including meat. Which do you think the body is better adapted to?

What does cooking do? It causes proteins to alter their structure, as can readily be seen when an egg turns opaque or a piece of meat turns brown. The amino acids of such proteins, which the body will use to build new bodily tissues, become damaged.

Some vitamins are destroyed or damaged, as well as certain phyto-chemicals. Fats become partially oxidized. But most of all, as we have seen, all the enzymes are destroyed. And various toxic compounds are created, among them radiolytic products (the same as are formed when a body is exposed to radiation).

A number of experiments have been performed on the effects of raw versus cooked food, beginning with Francis Pottenger's famous experiments on cats.

What Pottenger did was simplicity itself. He fed two groups of cats exactly the same diet, except that one group got it cooked and the other got it raw. Then he observed the results through four generations of cats.

The cooked-food cats developed various infections and degenerative diseases similar to those seen in human populations. After four generations the experiment had to be stopped since the cooked-food cats had died out. Meanwhile, those cats fed that same diet in a raw state continued to thrive and be healthy.

Why don't humans die out on a cooked-food diet? Probably because we don't eat an exclusively cooked diet. Our fresh fruit and salads and lightly cooked food (such as steaming or grilling) probably save us. Such raw or lightly-cooked foods enable the body to function, even when the situation is not ideal.

If we begin on a raw diet, we may not feel all the beneficial effects right away. Depending on how toxic the body is, we may feel worse instead of better for a time. This is so because a diet of living foods, like a fast, allows the body to accelerate its *detoxification* process.

CHAPTER 13

DETOXING

Each individual cell in the body is an unbelievably complex living organism in its own right. Each cell has many different sub-divisions of structure, and produces tens of thousands of different kinds of chemicals every day in the process of living.

Like all living things, the individual cell needs to take in nutrients to survive. It then releases energy from those nutrients, turns some of them into its own living structure, and also creates a product or service to export to the body as a whole, whether it be a hormone or a muscular contraction or a nerve impulse in the brain.

As part of this prodigious activity, the cell generates various toxic by-products, including highly reactive free radicals. These are sometimes called *endogenous wastes*, that is, wastes produced by the body itself.

The cell also has to contend with *exogenous wastes*, that is, toxins coming in from the outside. These include pesticides, food additives, pharmaceutical drugs, air and water pollution, heavy metals and PCBs in food, alcohol and fermented (partially decomposed) foods, excesses of protein and fat, recreational drugs and so on.

All toxic compounds must be rigorously removed from the cell if it is not to suffocate in its own waste. Meanwhile, the cell needs to continuously import oxygen and nutrients to continue its metabolism. Both of these functions are served by the *lymph fluid*.

The cell lives next to other cells in a sea of lymph fluid which contains both the nutrients the cell needs and the wastes which the cell has exported. The lymph fluid in turn is always near to a capillary of fast-moving blood which resupplies the lymph with nutrients and removes its accumulated wastes.

Experiments have shown that cells outside the body can be kept alive indefinitely if 1) they are fed the proper nutrients, and most important, 2) they are continually drained of wastes. Both are necessary.

Deficiency diseases are quite possible. Examples are the scurvy that British sailors suffered when denied access to fresh plant foods, or the multiple vitamin and mineral deficiencies in those who live on "empty calorie" diets of mostly refined foods, and which show up as problems of the eyes, nerves, skin, etc.

In industrialized societies, though, by far the more common problem is build-up of toxic wastes inside the cells of the body. The body has very efficient systems to clear itself of these toxins, but if the amount is too great the systems can become overloaded.

On the kinds of diets in industrialized societies, for instance, the body gets excess fat, protein, cholesterol and sodium, all of which must be dealt with as toxins. In the absence of sufficient unrefined carbohydrates, the body must burn protein or fat or both as fuel. This is a "dirty" process, akin to burning kerosene in your car, which creates many more toxic by-products.

And the body must deal with pesticides, additives, "empty-calorie" sugars and starches, dioxin, the damaged nutrients in cooked food, etc. All of this, continued over long periods of time, tends to overwhelm the eliminative systems. As this happens, first the lymph fluid and then the cells themselves become polluted.

As the toxic load of the cells increases, they become less efficient both in producing energy and in exporting their "product" to the body. Thus systems such as the immune or digestive or endocrine systems become less efficient and eventually begin to break down.

All of this is masked for awhile because the body makes heroic adjustments to operate under its toxic load. But when we don't eat for a couple of days, the actual state of things is revealed. We see it and feel it.

Why? Because when we stop eating, the digestive expenditure of the body is vastly reduced. Suddenly it does not have to digest all of the usual food.

A similar result occurs when we eat a fruitarian diet or a live food diet. The body finds that it expends much less energy to digest these foods. Fruit, for instance, is a clean-burning food which leaves few toxic by-products, and yet provides huge amounts of enzymes and phytochemicals.

Digestion takes more energy by far than any other process in the body. When the body expends less energy on digestion it has more vital power available to commit elsewhere—and begins to direct much more energy to its most important challenge, the build-up of pollutants and toxins in its cells and systems.

Thus the body begins a "spring cleaning" of sorts, pulling toxins out of the woodwork and directing them into the blood, from where they can be eliminated. But in the meantime we can feel miserable. More toxins are circulating in the bloodstream, the urine is turning dark with toxins, the breath becomes foul as toxins are eliminated by the lungs, we might have a runny nose as toxins are eliminated by mucous, and so forth.

This is a positive phenomenon, yet paradoxically we look and feel worse at first. We have less energy—the body is directing energy elsewhere—and/or we have the symptoms of a "cold" or "flu," etc.

And as a fast continues, various "healing crises" can occur as the body reaches deeper levels of toxins. This is balanced, however, by a distinct sense that one's overall well-being is increasing. Frequently, symptoms of long-standing conditions and diseases begin fading away. The effect is often quite amazing.

Indeed, fasting is the closest thing to a universal "miracle drug" on the physical level that I have ever come across. All kinds of ailments and illnesses and symptoms can begin to clear up on a fast, frequently without even having a diagnosis. It may not matter whether we know what's wrong—what matters is that the body knows, and goes to work on the matter.

Needless to say, on any fast whether short or long it is extremely valuable to get professional supervision from someone trained and experienced in fasting, so that your specific situation can be taken into account.

It's sometimes thought that fasting is equivalent to starvation, but that's not so. On a fast the body consumes itself in order to have nourishment, but in its wisdom it consumes dead cells, aged cells, diseased cells, etc. first, so that the overall effect is cleansing and renewal.

After the first few days of a fast the body turns off the appetite, signaling that it doesn't want us to eat for awhile so that it can stay focused on its cleansing. So in general, we don't walk around hungry on a fast. On the contrary, we usually feel a great freedom from hunger.

The Natural Way

As a fast continues into several weeks it becomes a spiritual journey as we begin to feel a surprising lightness and radiance inside. As the fast continues the tongue will become clear, the eyes will become bright, the skin will take on a healthy glow.

Sometime around 4 or 5 weeks usually, though it can vary a lot, the body suddenly turns the appetite back on. This is the body's signal that it has completed its process of detoxification for now, and that it wants us to eat again. This re-entry process to eating should be a gradual one, starting with juices or fruits and progressing slowly over several days to vegetables and grains and whatever else one is eating.

If we continue the fast beyond this signal of clean tongue and returning appetite, then we enter the process of starvation where the body is consuming its vital tissues to live. If we fast beyond this sign then we're starving and death comes in a couple more months or so.

Fasting, unlike starvation, is very beneficial to the body. Yet one fast, even a long one, may not be enough to clear the toxins from one's body. For most of us, toxemia has built up over decades, so it can take several years of a living food diet and periodic fasts to finish the process of cleansing. But that's okay; there's no rush.

What matters is allowing the body to begin.

CHAPTER 14

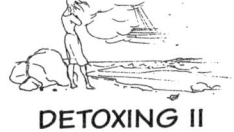

DETOXING II

What if, as a friend of mine said, we have to keep working at our jobs and don't have time to fast and rest right now? How to detox in that case?

In my opinion, the most useful step in any case is to move towards a live food diet. Such a diet is always detoxing. On a live food diet the body will not detox as rapidly or deeply as on a fast, yet it will clearly make a tremendous amount of progress in detoxifying.

And our diet need not be all live foods to benefit. Rather, the more we move *in the direction* of an uncooked diet, the more deeply and rapidly the body will detox itself. In the beginning, we can start with something as simple as just eating fruit and fresh-squeezed juice for breakfast instead of a cooked breakfast.

The Natural Way

Fruit is the most perfect food we can eat. It takes minimal energy to digest, thus allowing the body to use energy elsewhere, particularly in cleansing. Fruit provides high-quality, clean-burning energy surrounded by fiber and minerals and enzymes. It is alkalizing and leaves no residue in the body.

It's no accident that Dr. Walker found that we have been fruitarians for most of our existence.

In moving towards a cleansing diet, one successful method has been to start eating fruit for breakfast and then gradually extend this fruit-eating period to later and later in the day. Other ways of adding live foods are to eat more salads, more tomato or vegetable sandwiches, more raw corn on-the-cob, and so on.

I know some successful live food enthusiasts whose diet is over 90% fresh fruit. I know others, successful as well, who eat about 50-60% live food and add in things like baked potatoes and steamed vegetables. It's all up to each person. The Hunzas, by the way, get about 60% of their calories from raw foods, mainly fruit.

People with extensive experience in live food diets have found that raw nuts—which botanists classify as fruits—are very valuable on such a diet. When eaten in moderation, they add good quality protein and fat to the diet while preserving its live-food character. Leafy greens are also considered quite valuable in such diets for their phyto-chemicals.

Part of a successful detoxing program lies in getting enough sleep. It's during deep sleep at night that the body most effectively rebuilds and repairs and detoxes itself. During the inactivity of rest and sleep, the body is gaining vital strength and power. Eight hours is highly recommended, and more if one is healing.

How does detoxing affect weight loss? Notice, first of all, that animals in the wild, who eat live foods and have cleansed bodies, are never overweight. There are no overweight Hunzakuts. Adelle Davis pointed out that if we concentrate on *building health*, rather than losing weight, the body itself will take care of the weight.

The experience of the late T.C. Fry, a discerning health teacher, is fairly typical. When Fry began a live food diet he weighed 200 pounds and, at 5'5" in height, was quite overweight. On a live food diet he gradually lost weight and went down to just 126 pounds.

He was rather thin at this point and became a bit concerned for himself, but he kept on. And then something remarkable happened. *On the very same diet* he began to *gain weight* and then went up to 155 pounds, where he remained for the rest of his life.

What happened is that his body did a good detox and in that process went down to a minimum level. And then, the body having balanced itself and restored its energy and digestive efficiency, *it took itself* back to an ideal weight.

The Natural Way

So if we're challenged by obesity, we can shift our attention from the weight itself to *building our health*. As we do so, the body will normalize our weight just as it normalizes many other things.

If we're too thin, the same applies. For instance, we may be eating but not digesting food properly. When the organs of digestion and assimilation are given a relative rest, as they are on a live food diet, they usually become efficient once more, and then weight gain results.

Another thing that often shifts during a detox is mental health. As the body normalizes everything else, it also does its best to balance brain chemistry. People often notice restlessness, depression, etc. lifting naturally.

Sometimes it's said that we shouldn't eat fruit or raw vegetables because of candida or allergies or digestive problems and so on, but this is normally so only while the body is toxified. Once cleansed, the body usually handles all living fruits and vegetables with ease.

What about detoxing and water?

It's often repeated that we must "drink 8 glasses of water every day." But this requirement only applies when we're eating high-protein diets, since the metabolism of protein requires large amounts of water. On a live food diet, a great deal less water is required.

Raw, live fruits and vegetables are what is known as *high-water-content* foods. They are 80%-90% water, and on a live food diet often no other water is needed.

But even if it is, we can trust the body again and simply drink when we're thirsty, as nature intended. As we allow a more natural way into our life we find that we can trust that way more and more.

All other foods are *concentrated foods,* that is, they are low-water-content. All cooked food is concentrated. All animal foods are concentrated foods. Breads, pastas and so forth are all concentrated foods.

Anything that is concentrated has some addictive potential. Raw coca leaf, for example, is not addictive. But concentrated as cocaine, it is addictive. Concentrated further as crack cocaine, it's even more addictive.

But addictive substances aren't limited to drugs and alcohol. All concentrated foods also have some addictive potential. Thus meats, fats, sugar, salt and so on, being refined or concentrated, can all be considered somewhat addictive to us. And as with any addictive substance, when we eat such things we feel stimulated, we often "feel better" in some way temporarily.

But once the body is detoxified it does not need anything to feel good, nor does it feel better after food, since it already feels a remarkable sense of well-being in the first place.

Such a level of steady vitality and well-being, which can be quite surprising, is actually our natural state.

CHAPTER 15

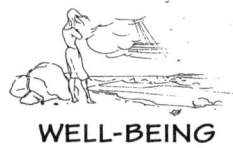
WELL-BEING

In 1822 a physician named Isaac Jennings came up with an interesting idea. He was not too thrilled with the treatments of his day, the bloodlettings and drug mercury treatments and so on. He noticed that his patients often got sicker, or died, on these treatments.

He became convinced that the body itself was the regenerative force, and that if the body was given a rest, in terms of both digestion and activity, that it could most readily heal itself. But he knew that his patients wanted drugs; they were convinced that something coming from the outside would heal them.

So Jennings mixed up some bread pills and colored water in bottles. These were pills and potions that would "do nothing." Then he told his patients that these special

Pt 2—Vitality

drugs did not go well with food, and that they needed to fast and rest for a week or two while taking them.

The result was miraculous. All manner of diseases were cured. In fact, Jennings became so popular that it was said no other physician could do business in the area around him.

After some years of this, Jennings decided to tell the truth about what he was doing, and that the real healer was the body, aided and abetted by "doing nothing." The result? He was denounced as a fraud and almost went out of business.

But meanwhile his friend Sylvester Graham caught the baton. Starting around 1831, Graham gave speeches to large crowds where he preached revolutionary ideas: That contrary to advice, fresh fruits and vegetables and fresh air were good for you, animal food and drugs made you toxic, flour should be whole-grain, and that cleanliness—both internal and external—was important.

The radical thing that Graham was saying was that health resulted not from pills, potions or various high- or low-tech treatments, but from making healthful choices every day. Rest, sleep, exercise when not fasting, fresh air, a live food diet, emotional poise and so on allowed the body to maximize its power to both maintain and restore organic balance and health in all areas of itself.

All the factors of a natural lifestyle were important, said Graham. Diet was given special prominence because

The Natural Way

it had been found on a practical basis to make the most difference—as McCarrison had also found.

From Graham, the physician Russell Trall caught the baton. Trall was the great systemizer of what he called *natural hygiene*. And he formulated this principle:

That the natural factors most useful in maintaining a state of health will be the most useful in allowing the body to heal itself when ill.

And conversely, those factors harmful to the body in a state of health will be harmful to it in a state of illness also. Only those substances which the body can use as *nutrients* are positive for the body, said Trall. The body must deal with all non-nutritive substances as toxins and expend energy to neutralize or expel them.

Picture yourself as a primate living perhaps a few million years ago in the African forest. You eat fruit and nuts and greens—whatever you can easily gather in the trees and near them. Your food is naturally fresh, living, vegetarian, low-fat, unprocessed, enzyme-rich.

You have no drugs, potions, magnets or electrical devices; no doctors, nobody to adjust anything. You have nothing to cook with. You have no way of knowing how often or on what schedule you should eat—that depends on the food supply. You have no knowledge of any blood type. You have no weight scale.

Pt 2—Vitality

Yet nature has designed you so that, barring a serious accident, you will remain illness-free all your life—as animals in the wild do and as Hunzas, Vilcabambans and others do today.

Imagining when and how we lived in the wild can answer many questions in a practical way. Such as: What should we eat to be truly healthy?

Let's rephrase that question:

What foods would we be attracted to in the wild?

Would we bite into an apple? Of course. Would we bite into a raw garlic or ginger? Probably not. So that lets us know that such foods are probably best used in small quantities if at all.

Would we need to know about any "magic foods" to stay healthy? No, we wouldn't need to get bee pollen or brewer's yeast or fiber in a can. We wouldn't need a protein drink or the latest vitamin or prescription drug or herbal remedy. Yet we'd be superbly healthy.

Would a steak be available to us a few million years ago when we lived in the trees? How about a peach pie, canned vegetables, cheese? No. What would be available is what we know as *fresh produce* in the market. When we ingest living, unprocessed, plant-based foods we're eating as nature intended. And the body responds.

The body is a self-generating, self-maintaining and self-healing organism, said Trall, *and it is the only healing power there is.*

The Natural Way

No drug, no herb can act upon the body to heal it; these are inactive, non-living substances. Only the body has the *vital power* to act, and it heals itself when it is intelligently left alone.

If an animal sustains a serious wound, it goes off by itself somewhere and does not eat, but just rests for as long as necessary. When we go to a health center and fast and rest under supervision we're essentially doing the same thing. The Natural Hygiene pioneers like Jennings and Trall spoke of "doing nothing" and allowing the body to exercise its innate, natural, healing intelligence.

The body is striving at all times to reach the highest harmony possible for itself. When we're ill, therefore, we supply a fast and/or natural diet, fresh air and water, moderate sunlight, lots of rest, relaxing thoughts, etc., but otherwise do nothing.

In other words, *we supply the conditions for health* and the body heals itself using its own vital power.

Health comes from healthy living.

Health comes from supplying the conditions for health—that is, from focusing on causes rather than trying to get rid of symptoms. Instead of suppressing the symptoms of a headache or "cold," we allow the body to detox and redress the imbalance that is causing it.

What we sow, we reap. Diseases don't just show up out of nowhere, the pioneers of natural hygiene saw. Illness is caused by a gradual enervation of the body's vital power—which shows up in specific areas—either brought on by a lack of nutrients or, more likely, by the gradual accumulation of a toxic load which impedes the body's functioning.

The body works at all times to excrete toxins, but over time it can become overwhelmed because it wasn't designed to deal with the kinds and amounts of toxins presented to it by high-protein, high-fat diets, cooked and chemicalized foods, pesticides, etc. And it detoxes as much as it can, but then the next such meal comes down, and the next... The body begins to fall behind in its detoxing efforts, and this can go on for decades.

This inner pollution can show up as arterial plaque that narrows arteries, raising blood pressure; it can show up in the joints as calcium crystals; it can show up in the cells as free radicals—and many other ways and places. But what this toxicity really means, however or wherever it shows up, is a *generalized* enervation of the body, which shows up as various kinds of symptoms.

Drugs, herbs, electrical and other stimulations and so on can suppress the symptoms of this toxemia, but fundamentally do not get at the cause of it. Taking drugs and so on to suppress the symptoms increases the body's poisoning and thus, long-term, *increases* the symptoms.

CHAPTER 16

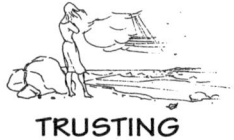

TRUSTING

Herbert Shelton, who caught the natural hygiene baton from Trall in the 20th century, pointed out that for every drug or manipulation used on the body there is a *primary effect* and a *secondary effect*.

The primary effect is the obvious one, the one that works on the symptom. For example, let's say we feel a bit lethargic and we want a boost in energy. We take some substance that makes us feel stimulated, such as a cup of coffee or some cocaine. And we do feel more energetic, more "invigorated" for the moment.

But then the law of compensation comes into play. The extra energy produced by the body has to come from somewhere, and so after the stimulation then a period of greater lethargy than before occurs.

Continued over time, the secondary effect, *which is the exact opposite of the primary effect,* becomes more and more pronounced.

The drug or herb we take to stimulate us gradually exhausts us. The drug we take to calm us gradually makes us more tense. The substance we take to lift our mood gradually depresses it.

For instance, in the beginning a shot of heroin is very relaxing. But over time the body actually builds up more restlessness because of it.

This is revealed if we try to do without the heroin for two days. Then, as we're going through hell detoxing, our true state is revealed as extreme restlessness—and it's the exact opposite of what we took the heroin for in the first place, to seek relaxation. The secondary effect gradually supercedes the primary one.

When we have an infection, the body itself creates the fever because the immune system is more efficient at higher temperatures. Then when we take something to lower the fever (unless it's life-threatening), we're actually working against the body's efforts, and thus prolonging the illness of which the fever is a symptom.

When we have a "cold" or "flu," actually symptoms of a toxic body, the body itself produces the runny nose and coughing as an emergency attempt to excrete its toxic overload. Pathogenic organisms are always around. What really matters is the soil those seeds are falling on—how vital is the body? When we take something to stop the runny nose, etc., we're actually making the job of the body—*the only healer*—more difficult.

The problem is almost never truly external. A body that is healthy easily throws off all manner of parasites and pathogens. A body that is fully detoxed just doesn't get "colds" and "flus" and "allergies" and low-energy and other toxic signs. But it can be difficult to believe this until we experience it for ourselves.

When we use drugs or other processes to suppress the symptoms of a disease, then, we're actually working against our own body. We're suppressing the symptom—that's the primary effect—but long-term we're increasing the disease—the secondary effect.

The very chemotherapy that eliminates a tumor—that's the primary effect—severely damages the immune system also and greatly increases the body's toxic load, thus tending to promote a more generalized cancer later on. That's the secondary effect, the hidden effect.

When we take antacids to neutralize acidity in the stomach, the body produces *more* acid long-term in order to counteract the effects of the antacids. The secondary effect gradually supersedes the primary effect.

Every force we try to impose upon the body produces its opposite effect long-term. Everything we take to "sustain," "invigorate" or "stimulate" the body actually lowers its strength and works against its healing.

Conversely, when we're resting and detoxing and looking weak, the body is gaining power to the greatest extent possible.

According to Shelton, the body can be trusted to make the wisest allocation of its own resources. The body is not lazy; it doesn't need a little jogging to make it do the right thing. On the contrary, the body knows everything about itself and is always allocating resources in the highest, best possible way.

Thus we supply the body with the natural nutrients it needs, avoid giving it anything else, avoid trying to manipulate it, and give it a deep rest both digestively and physically. Then the body itself does the rest.

All drugs and other agents are attempts to stimulate or suppress one or more of the body's systems. They try to push the body in a certain direction. Yet the body itself knows how best to direct its energies and is doing so at all times. Attempts to manipulate this process only impede its efforts.

Hence Jennings' description of resting, fasting, and "doing nothing" as the greatest assistance to the body's healing. They support the body's own vital power, and do nothing to interfere with it.

Shelton supervised over 40,000 fasts in his lifetime, and came to feel that interventions of any kind were misguided. Even enemas, for instance, though "cleansing" on the surface, created a secondary effect of lax bowels. The body was capable, he saw, of cleaning out an intestine just as much as an artery or anything else, and didn't benefit from any forcing efforts. He noticed that fasting patients did best when they took no heroic measures, and just let nature have its own timetable. Non-interference.

It's sometimes said that while fasting we need to take honey and lemon juice, or bentonite clays, or special herbs or juices or fruits, etc. to "stimulate" cleansing.

But Shelton observed that the body needed no stimulation for this, that at all times it was cleansing and rebalancing in the most efficient way possible. He saw that all so-called aids and stimulants to that process were just more toxins or stresses that the body needed to deal with, thus *slowing down* the overall healing process.

Building on Trall, Shelton espoused the view that all drugs were lifeless, inert agents that had no power to act in the body. Rather, that the "effects" of drugs were actually *the body's actions* to neutralize or expel the poison or irritation that was being encountered.

Given a diuretic, the body increases fluid flowing from the kidneys to more quickly expel the irritant. With laxatives, the body creates diarrhea to more quickly expel the poison. With "stimulants," the body rises to a higher state of activity temporarily to counter the toxins.

In all cases it's *the body itself that is acting*. Only life has the power to act; the drug or treatment has no power to do anything.

Since the body has to expend energy to respond to all such things, long-term they impede the body's efforts and increase its overall enervation. The wisest course, said Shelton, is to trust the body's innate intelligence, which knows what to do far better than we do.

Yet absolutist positions are not warranted. There is a place for all things at one time or another. Supplements can be helpful in deficiencies. Drugs and procedures can save our lives in emergencies and epidemics. I once threw out my back and was very glad to see a chiropractor. Many other examples could be given.

But in general, we're wise to respect the body and its great inherent power, to support its efforts and avoid various attempts to manipulate it—to see that only the body itself can heal itself permanently, and needs no stimulation or outside force in order to do so.

Our efforts need not be all-or-nothing; no need to be fanatical. We don't need to be full-on raw-foodists or vegetarians, for example, to benefit from these notions.

Every time we eat a living food instead of a cooked one, a peach instead of a peach pie, a starch instead of a steak, a salad instead of canned vegetables, organic foods instead of irradiated, altered or pesticided foods and so on—we're supporting the body.

Every time we allow the body to cleanse instead of further toxifying, every time we eat a living, organic food, we're supporting the body's own natural efforts.

The Natural Way

A natural lifestyle supportive to the body can be very enjoyable and approached in a relaxing way. While at first the idea of a living food or vegan diet can seem radical, with time we actually come to prefer them. In my experience, this usually takes about four months.

It can be very simple. For example: Fresh fruit for breakfast; a vegetable sandwich and coleslaw for lunch; burritos with mostly raw ingredients for dinner. There are infinite possibilities. A number of quite good vegan and live food recipe books are appearing on the market now and are well worth exploring.

When contemplating new life paths, it's wise to get professional assistance. No path on this earth is riskless, and so experienced professional advice, *which can take our personal situation into account*, is priceless.

For more information on the topics discussed here, a good place to begin would be the American Natural Hygiene Society in Tampa, FL, 813-855-6607, or Living Nutrition in Sebastopol, CA at 707-887-9132.

Using insight, we can let a path of greater vitality and aliveness express in our life by living closer to nature and the natural way of things. Then the Energy moves through us at the bodily level, as in other dimensions of our life, and we tend to unfold more and more into the graceful harmony of our true nature.

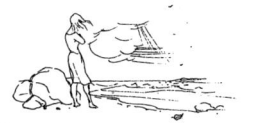

PART 3
Freedom

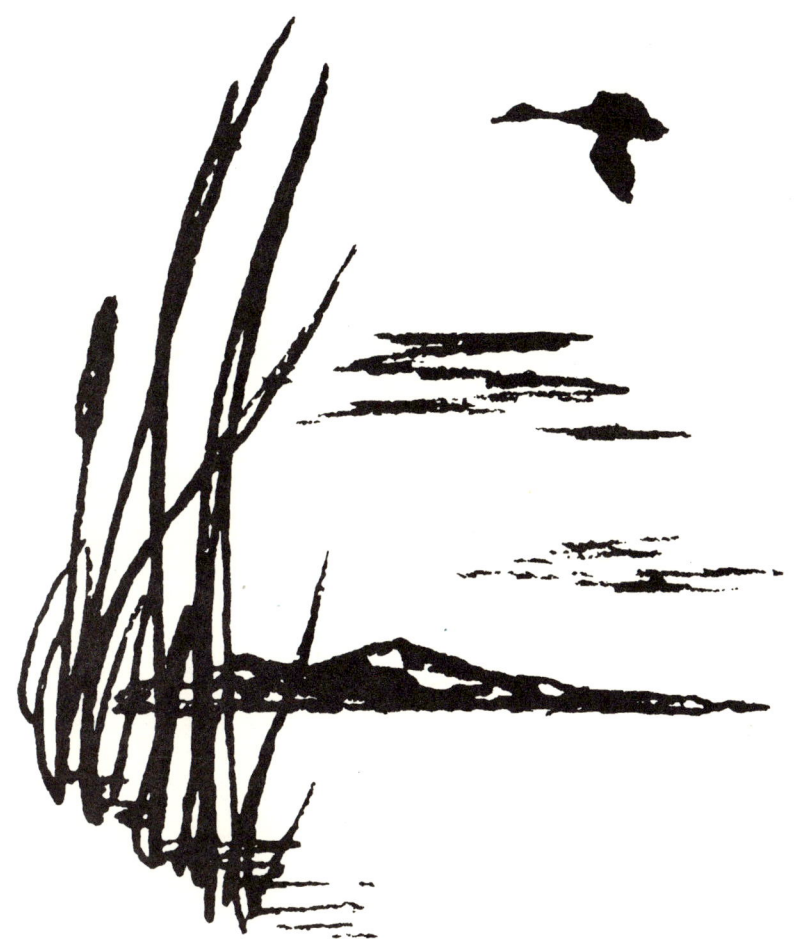

CHAPTER 17

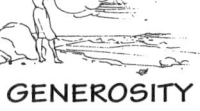

GENEROSITY

Each of us has a unique path in life. No one else's answers can truly be our answers. Only the answer that comes from within ourselves can truly be ours.

The Buddha said that 2500 years ago, and added, "Be a lamp unto yourselves." Jesus said, "The kingdom of heaven is within you." They and other great teachers seem to be pointing to something inside us as holding the natural key to life's mystery and meaning.

To convey what is found there, various mystical traditions have used a metaphor about the shining of the sun. When it's a cloudy day we sometimes say that the sun isn't shining. Yet if we climb a mountain or take a plane above the clouds, we immediately see that the sun is there, it's shining, and has always been shining.

The Natural Way

That metaphor, the mystics say, is approximately our situation. We have a kind of sun shining inside of us, a warm, bright, loving intelligence that is always shining, but yet is obscured by clouds.

Those clouds, they say, are formed by our thoughts and images and desires and emotions and aversions and so on. All of that together is our "cloudy sky."

They also point out that it's not necessary to do anything about the sun. Rather, that once the clouds are no longer obscuring the sky, that the natural luminosity of our essential nature reveals itself inherently.

If *Part 1–Happiness* is grounded in the teachings of Jesus, then *Part 3–Freedom* is grounded in the teachings of the Buddha, though it also includes other teachers and personal experience.

The Buddha was very brilliant and compassionate, but also quite practical—he was interested in showing us how to do things. This Part 3, then, attempts to embody that down-to-earth emphasis.

Those in all ages who have gone within invite us to do it too and find for ourselves our essential nature. And they promise that if we do, it will transform our life.

These words are about that inner journey.

It's a journey that I'm travelling also. In part these words are for my own sake, to increase my own clarity in taking this journey myself. And I'd love it if these words could somehow benefit you.

The Buddha suggested beginning the inner journey with the cultivation of the quality of *generosity*, and then what he called the *precepts*.

And he gave a very interesting reason for following these suggestions for outer behavior. Because following these "skillful means," as he called them, would tend to quiet down the stormiest or most cloudy waves of the mind and thus be very helpful to our journey inward.

He pointed out that if we're acting unethically, or "unskillfully" as he said, our journey within will be very difficult because the mind will be too agitated or numbed out. So these are measures taken in everyday life that allow the mind to find the beginnings of peace.

Generosity is cultivated as a kind of training wheels for the mind. It's a good antidote to the mind's usual tendency to cling—to objects, beliefs, desires, stories about other people, etc. This clinging tendency was identified by the Buddha as the root cause of suffering.

Generosity reverses the flow of our mind's clinging and grasping. When we look for ways to be generous, we immediately increase our own sense of well-being and happiness. Generosity tends to open up the mind's sense of tightness, allowing it to begin to relax.

So, to begin, we can practice giving to others. This can range from doing a favor to saying a kind word. A great sense of lightness comes over us when we begin to look for ways to be generous without thought of return.

The Natural Way

It's a great paradox, too, but the more valuable the things that we give away—"Oh no, I couldn't give *that* away"—the lighter we feel.

Being generous to others also means adopting a non-harming attitude towards them, and here we'll talk about the precepts.

Later on, when the mind begins to open to its own luminosity, our actions will be a spontaneous and unique intuitively moral response to each situation. It will naturally tend towards the most harmonious outcome for all concerned. But for now we cultivate skillful actions to reduce impediments to the mind's inward journey.

The first precept is not to physically harm others, that is, not to kill them, strike them and so on. Such unskillful actions create great turmoil.

The second precept is not to steal from others—that is, not to take from somebody or an organization something that hasn't been offered, or hasn't been offered in the way that we're thinking of taking it.

The third precept is not to be unskillful in speaking with others. This includes following our inner truth in saying "yes" or "no," avoiding harsh and unkind speech to others, and avoiding untruthful speech, all of which feed the mind's tendency to tighten.

The fourth precept concerns the sexual and romantic area. Since this is such a strong drive, the tendency to manipulate others in this area is strong. We act skillfully in this area by avoiding manipulations of others and by respecting their right to whatever boundaries they deem appropriate.

The basic thrust of these precepts is to put into practice Jesus' Golden Rule—that is, to treat others as we would like them to treat us.

The fifth precept is to avoid intoxicants of various kinds, everything from nicotine to alcohol to uppers and downers and hallucinogens, anything that can cloud the mind and reduce its essential brightness. We could say that this is going for a different kind of "high," what we might call a Clarity High.

The initial purpose of these actions, again, is for our own sake—to reduce as much as possible actions that tend to greatly disturb or cloud the mind and thus reduce its capacity to undertake the inward journey.

CHAPTER 18

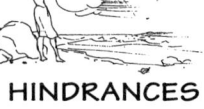

HINDRANCES

Next we become aware of what are known as the *hindrances*, that is, states of mind that disturb the mind's essential luminosity, both in everyday life and in sitting meditation.

We accept these hindrances to whatever extent that they're there, but we begin to pay attention. We begin to notice how they disturb the mind's essential stability and peace. Over time, in doing this, we develop a natural equanimity towards these states of mind; that is, we can watch them without feeling that we need to act on them. We begin to see the robotic nature of the hindrances.

The first is *greed*, which can come in various hues, whether for money or power or sensuality or the desire to be right. It's not that we reject greed or any of the other hindrances—they'll come up whenever they do—but we begin to watch them rather than act them out. This hindrance of greed can be compared to water in which a red dye has been placed. Even a relatively small amount of dye can render opaque a large amount of water and prevent the observer from seeing to the stillness of the bottom.

The second hindrance is the opposite of the first, that is, *aversion* of various kinds. This includes when our mind goes to places of ill-will, anger, hatred, irritation, discontent and so on. Again, we don't try to repress these feelings, but we do bring attention to them; we begin to notice how they deeply unsettle the mind. In that very noticing, they begin to gradually become more flimsy.

This hindrance has been compared to water that is boiling, and thus opaque in that way to seeing down into the depths of the water.

The third hindrance is *laziness and dullness*. Here we notice the mind's tendency sometimes to fall into a state of numbness, where it doesn't want to notice the reality of what is going on inside. The mind distracts itself in various ways—anything from zealotry to drugs to shopping to TV to compelling ideas will do—and thus dulls itself in a kind of sleepiness, so that it cannot perceive its inherent warm and loving brightness. So we begin to notice the times when we've dulled ourselves in some way.

The Natural Way

This hindrance has been compared to water overgrown by weeds and algae, so that once again the depths of the water cannot be seen.

The fourth hindrance is the opposite of the third, that is, *restlessness* in its different forms, which includes worry and agitation and fear. Again, it's not that we try to repress restlessness or fear when it appears, but we do begin to notice the mind's tendency to go there when it imagines that things or situations or people have to be a certain way that *it* thinks is best.

When we judge that someone should be different then we're in their business instead of our own—and we begin to notice how we suffer when we get into someone else's business.

This hindrance has been compared to water that is swept by fierce winds, so that the water is no longer transparent and naturally clear.

The fifth hindrance is *skeptical doubt,* which can prevent us from undertaking any worthwhile path of growth. This usually takes two forms: One is nihilism—"This world is illusory and empty and nothing matters, so there's no point in exerting myself."

The other pole of doubt is externalism—"All these glittering objects in the world exist independently and are the real source of happiness, so I'll just devote myself to grasping and indulging in them. What's the point of looking into my inner world?"

This hindrance has been compared to water that is in darkness, so that once again the depths of it cannot be observed and experienced.

These hindrances were set out by the Buddha many years ago, but they are equally relevant now because awareness of them is still very conducive to seeing how the mind disturbs its essential peace.

When the hindrances arise, we just let them settle down by letting them be there and shifting to watching them instead of grabbing them and acting on them. It's kind of like sitting on the bank of a muddy pond and watching the mud naturally settle by itself.

CHAPTER 19

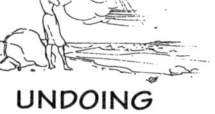

UNDOING

The third facet of this inward journey, in my opinion, is the work of the teacher Byron Katie.

It might seem strange that right in the middle of the Buddha's insights I start talking about Byron Katie. But I'd be remiss if I didn't. Of all the many approaches to personal development that I've looked into, Katie's seems to me the simplest and yet the most profound. To me it seems an indispensable tool in helping to undo the mind and thus to facilitate the journey within.

My description of Katie's work is just my personal understanding, so you may want to contact her center directly to hear a tape or attend a gathering. In addition, Katie has sheets and booklets to assist with the process of The Work, and they can also be obtained by contacting

Pt 3—Freedom

The Work Foundation at www.thework.org or at (760) 256-5653 in Barstow, CA.

The Work begins by writing down something that bothers or upsets us. We write it down to stop the mind, to photograph it for a moment so that we can better work with it. In doing this we allow that petty, judgmental part of us to fully express. As Katie says, we've been instructed for years not to judge, and it's still what we do best.

Thus we drop for a moment any spiritual insights that we may have picked up, and let ourselves really feel and express the hurt child inside.

Experienced students of the Work sometimes just write down their stream-of-thought about something that's bothering them, and begin the Inquiry right from there. Katie provides sheets to assist in writing down our complaints in a more structured form, asking ourselves questions such as:

Concerning this person or situation, what is it that's bothering me? How should they or it be different? What do I want them to do? What are my opinions of them? What is it I don't ever want to experience again?

In writing these things, we deliberately project our attention outside—that is, we judge our neighbor or some situation rather than ourselves. The reason for this will become evident a little later.

Once we have our upset feelings written down in a series of statements, we then begin to investigate those

The Natural Way

statements. Basically, we inquire about their truthfulness and their effects upon us.

So we ask ourselves inside, "Is this belief true? Can I really know that it's true?" When we go within and really look at the belief we discover that we can't be certain of it and that no belief or story is really true. Every belief is just a story of some kind that we've got going and that we've velcroed to.

Then we ask ourselves the question, "What do I get from holding this belief?" And variations of it, such as: How do I live when I hold this belief? How do I treat myself and others when I hold it? Can I see a reason to hold onto it other than suffering?

When we really look inside we find that holding on to the belief is causing us misery and suffering and feelings of isolation and separation. We see that clearly, we feel it acutely.

Then we look at the other side, the positive side: "Who would I be without this belief?" How would I act, how would I live? When we really look, we usually find that without the belief we would be much more free and available, much more open and joyful.

It can have a powerful effect to look at the truth of our stories and then examine the costs of holding on to them and the benefits of letting go.

But then Katie gives us the kicker; she has us reverse everything. Every statement that we've written down, we turn it around. If we've written down, "Ellen is insensitive towards me," we turn it around to, "I am insensitive towards Ellen."

And then we really look inside to see if we can find the turn-around. We look to see if the reversal statement isn't at least as true as the original one.

And it's the most amazing thing—when we truly look, we find that we've been doing to the other what we've accused them of doing to us. Sometimes we've been doing it overtly, and sometimes just in our mind.

Let's take an example: A friend called the other day and said that her fiance was "too much in his head" and "hasn't made love to me in weeks."

The first statement, turned around, became "I am too much in my head." She had the courage to look at that, and found it: She *was* too much in her head lately, especially when she was judging her fiance to be too much in his head.

Then she turned around the second statement and it became, "I haven't made love to him in weeks." This puzzled her; she couldn't find it. Then I asked her if she had made love to her fiance in her mind lately, that is, had she been kind to him in her mind?

And then she found it. Yes, she had been very unkind toward him lately in her mind, criticizing and judging him a lot. So, really, she had not been making love to him lately. The turn-around was true.

Then she turned it around again. "I have not been making love to myself lately." She saw how true that was, how harsh she'd been with herself lately, and she cried.

When she saw this and some other things she lightened up tremendously, and suddenly felt a great sense of compassion towards her fiance—and herself. That is the power of Katie's work.

The purpose of these questions and turn-arounds isn't to whitewash anything, but to clearly see that the universe comes in dualities, and that what we accuse others of doing we're doing ourselves. If I think someone is being arrogant, *I'm* being arrogant in the very moment of judging them that way. To see this is very freeing.

Fundamentally, other people don't cause us to feel anything. If we didn't have a particular quality ourselves, we would have no emotional charge upon that quality in someone else. We might notice it, we might even think it fascinating, but we would not be disturbed by it.

For instance, let's suppose we're upset that "Joe is such an angry person." We see that it's *our* unconscious pool of anger—probably picked up in childhood and repressed—that is being denied and projected out.

In this example, Joe is doing or saying whatever he does or says. It's our mind that judges that wrong, or says that it shouldn't be that way, as if we know God's business better than God, as if the universe ought to conduct itself according to *our* ideas of how it should be.

In this example, if we didn't have that deep pool of unconscious anger in ourselves, we wouldn't have any particular charge on Joe's anger. We wouldn't have any energy on it; it would just be a fact.

The clue that something within ourselves is being stimulated by Joe is that we have an emotional charge about it. Then we know that it's not Reality but our disagreement with Reality that's causing us to suffer.

Reality is just the way it is. When we're in disagreement with Reality, we suffer. And it's our own disavowed quality inside that is causing us to suffer, in this case the anger we feel that's being generated internally but, we say, "caused" by Joe.

We look and see the truth—that we're causing our experience of Reality ourselves. Our internal experience is being self-generated based on past traumas and conditionings. It's stimulated by external events but not caused by them.

Here we're looking at the truth of our projections upon the world and other people. And because the world is just a big mirror to us, we understand who it is that we're really seeing and describing in our story. The only person we ever really see or describe is ourselves. What we see in others exists in us.

Then, the very thing that we said we weren't willing to experience again, we say that we *are willing* to experience it again. We say that and open to it. "I'm will-

The Natural Way

ing to experience this again," because it almost certainly will happen again—only this time we want to respond to it in a more open and transparent way.

And then we say and feel, "I *look forward* to experiencing this again." That final statement releases our grip on the story even more.

In my experience, Katie's work opens us up like nothing else. There are many, many valuable body-mind approaches out there, and I honor them all and have received benefit from many of them. I emphasize Katie's work because it's brilliant and deep and has great compassion as well. In my opinion, we're fortunate to have her on the planet.

CHAPTER 20

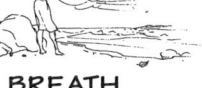
BREATH

Another aspect of the inward journey is to begin to deliberately cultivate profound states of concentration of the body-mind, both for their relaxing effect and also to prepare the mind for insight meditation.

This is done by refining concentration into a meditation, also known as tranquillity meditation.

Concentration is something that we all partake of to some extent. When we're focused on writing a term paper, making love or accomplishing a goal at work, we're partaking of the rudimentary stages of concentration meditation. But now we deliberately focus and intensify this effect.

In concentration meditation we focus the mind on a single point of attention and return it there again and again. The mind doesn't want to do this at first, because it's accustomed to roaming around at will. Our normal waking mind is compared in some traditions to a drunken monkey swinging chaotically through the trees. Now we're going to focus.

Often, when beginning concentration meditation, the mind will seem even more restless than usual. It's not, but in attempting to focus the mind on one point we'll begin to see just how restless our mind really is. Because it will go away to other things again and again. And each time we notice that, we can just gently return attention back to the concentration object.

One of the benefits of concentration is that by and by the mind will actually come into the present moment, as the organism slows down. More and more, the mind will be able to put down temporarily its burden of thoughts and judgments and cravings and conditionings—and the suffering they bring.

In concentration meditation, the mind's thoughts and conditionings are temporarily swept aside so that the mind can experience its innate spaciousness and brightness. When we stop doing the meditation, though, we come down from this "high."

But while its effects are temporary, concentration nevertheless is highly valuable both for giving a taste of what true liberation would actually be like, and also as a powerful tool for the next stage.

Our concentration object can be various things. It can be a *mantra*, for instance—a word or phrase such as "Rama" or "Allah" or "O Gracious God, have mercy on me," or "May all beings be happy" or "Om Mane Padme Hum" (the jewel in the lotus). I've tried these and other mantras from different traditions and found all of them to be effective.

Another possibility is a visual image of some kind. A *mandala* is such a visual image, usually of circles within circles. A *kasina* is a colored disc about the size of a dinner plate that one focuses on. Other examples could be a candle flame, a flower, the picture of one's guru or of someone who especially inspires us. The latter will arouse devotion, adding to the concentration.

One can also concentrate on a kinesthetic motion, such as Sufi whirling or rocking one's arm or body back and forth.

But having tried these and others, I have to admit to a bias in the end, because in my experience nothing compares with using the breath as one's object of concentration.

It's not an accident that the mystical tradition of virtually every spiritual path has some emphasis upon the breath—because the breath is so fundamental to us, it's so natural to our life as human beings.

The breath has many great qualities as a concentration object. First, it is always available under all circumstances. We are breathing from the moment we are born to the moment we die.

Second, it does not give rise to any hindrances, or emotional imbalances. Concentration upon things such as piling up money or power can lead to disturbances of the mind. Some phrases—examples might be "I am all-powerful" or "Death cannot touch me"—could also give rise to disturbances in the mind.

A third advantage of the breath is that it has no concepts associated with it. It's a purely natural process, part of nature, associated with the present moment rather than any concepts. The Buddha, who was among other things a consummate concentration master, chose the breath as his own object of concentration.

A final advantage to using the breath is that, unlike some other objects, it can lead to the highest states of concentration—what are known as the *jhanas,* or states of profound absorption.

We begin, normally, by sitting down. We can also lie down, but the risk of that position is sleepiness. We want to stay quite awake, so normally we sit up.

Sitting can be done on a cushion or in a chair.

On a cushion sitting can be done in the classic lotus or half-lotus posture, or in other positions where the legs are folded more casually. Or we can sit in a chair. The more we sit up straight in the chair, the more awake we'll tend to be.

The idea is just that we want to get into a position where we can remain stable and awake for a period of time. If we have to shift positions frequently, our meditation will suffer. The calmer and more stable our body is, the calmer and more stable the mind will be.

For the purposes of sitting meditation, a place that is quiet and undisturbed is ideal. We want to remove, as far as possible, all sources of distraction, so we can concentrate all our attention on the meditation object.

It's good to determine the length of the meditation before we go into it. If we leave it up to our whims, we tend to have short sessions because the mind will supply reasons to end the session prematurely. A timer is helpful since it's distracting to keep glancing at a watch.

To begin with, 20 or 30 minutes is good. Even 10 minutes will be beneficial. Over several months we can work up to sessions of an hour. A nice rhythm is to do half an hour in the morning and half an hour after work or before sleep. Experienced meditators often work three or four hours of meditation into their daily activities.

Normally we close our eyes. But we can do it with eyes open too. In that case we simply let our eyes gaze on a floor or wall a few feet in front of us, but without focusing on anything in particular.

Now we just watch the breath with our attention as it flows in and out. We watch the breath flow into our bodies and we watch it flow out of them without trying

The Natural Way

to control it in any way. This is not about breath control, but about watching without interference.

As we just watch our breath, it will naturally slow down and become calmer and more stable. This process calms the sympathetic nervous system (the fight or flight system) and promotes the parasympathetic nervous system instead (the relaxing and calming system).

To increase our concentration further, we want to sharpen our focus. We do this by fixing our attention upon the breath at a specific area.

One possibility is to use the rising and falling of the belly (*hara* in Zen) for this purpose. As the breath goes in, the belly rises; as it goes out, the belly falls. We can observe this rising and falling with our attention.

That is a good choice, and I worked with it for a long time. We often hold much of our unconscious tension in our bellies, and one of the advantages of focusing in this area is the reduction of that tension. Watching the breath at the belly is profoundly relaxing and can serve as a good anchor when we begin insight meditation, discussed a bit later.

But the object I have come to favor is the one most likely used by the Buddha himself, that is, watching the breath where it first comes into the body, at the nose.

When we take a breath, the air first strikes our nostrils at a certain point. For most people this point is at the inside tip of the nose, though for some it will be near the upper lip. We can experiment for ourselves: Take a few deep breaths through your nose and see where the initial sensation of the breath is most prominent.

This point where the breath is first noticed is called the *phusana*, the contact point. We now focus our attention there, watching the breath at that point.

In doing so, we emulate a gatekeeper. A gatekeeper lets people in or out, but doesn't follow them once they've passed the gate. In similar fashion, we watch the breath at the nose but no longer follow it into the body. We want to sharply focus our attention, and for that purpose the breath at the tip of the nose is ideal.

An amazing thing happens when we watch our breath in this way. Over time the breath becomes alive. It always was, of course, but we didn't notice it before. Now we're studying it, not by thinking about it, but directly, just watching it intently.

The breath has a lot to teach us about the cycles of life. We cannot have only in-breaths or only out-breaths, but must have both. As we watch the breath, it teaches us much about the dual nature of Existence, how the leaves and roots of the tree always exist together, how pleasure and pain, winning and losing must both be there.

But beyond that, the breath at this sharply focused point becomes a doorway into another dimension, the dimension of the present moment, the dimension where all true spiritual journeys begin.

As we meditate in this way, our attention will be distracted countless times onto other things. We become distracted by a thought and follow it and it turns into another and another. Seconds or minutes later we notice that and, using mindful awareness, return our attention to the breath.

As we continue in this way, our meditation slowly deepens. We get distracted less often, and for shorter times. Our breath becomes more vivid, more present and alive. We begin to feel a sense of merging with it.

CHAPTER 21

LIGHT

As our concentration practice deepens, the mind settles down and begins to take a quiet joy in itself. We begin to experience the mind's essential nature as being bliss when it isn't burdened down by incessant thinking and painful feelings, by craving and aversion.

When the mind is well concentrated these things are temporarily suppressed from consciousness and so the mind gets a glimpse of its true, spacious nature.

But concentration meditation does not extinguish these things. Our stories and cravings and resentments and so on simply go to the unconscious and bide their time. Then, when our concentration meditation is over, they slowly return to consciousness. The taste of our true nature is temporary.

Nevertheless, this daily concentration on the breath accomplishes a great deal. The body-mind begins to relax on a deep level that's not really reached by anything else. You'll find that you're less reactive in your daily life, that you have more of a sense of humor, that you're more easy-going. You'll find that your interactions with people tend to be more harmonious, and that you tend to enjoy life more. You'll notice these things and more.

These tendencies are especially so if to some extent we continue to focus on our breath as we go about our daily life. Not a big deal, but just a sort of background awareness of our breath at the contact point as we listen and cook and work and so on. From time to time we'll recollect ourselves, and let some of our attention return to our breath as we go about our business.

As we quiet down a little inside, our intuition becomes greater. Not only do we find that we can trust life more and more, but that our intuitive sense of how to function effectively in various situations increases.

There's an inner knowing inside each of us, a warm, bright, loving intelligence—beneath the level of thoughts and beliefs and cravings—that has a great sense of how to act and what to do in our lives.

As meditation deepens, we find ourselves hearing this "inner guidance" more and listening to it and acting upon it more. And listening less to the craziness of our ordinary mind.

Pt 3—Freedom

Any serious meditator sooner or later comes face to face with an astonishing realization: That his or her mind is completely crazy—that it's a chaotic, out-of-control bus careening madly down a steep hill with no brakes. It's always been that way, but we hadn't noticed it before because we were so caught up in it. Now we do notice, and it's a sobering moment when we really see it.

As meditators, as we become more relaxed we also become more tuned in to this inner guidance in our daily life. Whereas the thoughts of our ordinary mind tend to come from a need to feel safe, the intuitive wisdom of our inner guide comes from a different place.

Our inner guidance comes from a place of great love and possibility. As we quiet down a bit inside, this inner knowing, this warm bright intelligence within us begins to direct our activities more and we find that we're spontaneously doing things without knowing why sometimes. But we're following our own inner truth more.

Not that it's always a picnic. Oftentimes my inner guide or intelligence has suggested something to which my rational mind reacts, "Whoa! That's crazy! I can't do that!" But increasingly I've just gone ahead and followed it anyway, and almost always things have turned out in fulfilling ways that I couldn't have imagined from my rational mind.

Another way of saying this is that as our trust in life increases, we open up more to whatever wants to happen.

The Natural Way

We become more available to the Mystery of life and so more of that Mystery reveals Itself in our life.

It can seem pretty silly at times, I know, to sit there and watch our breath. The mind may remark what a silly thing it is, especially when we could be playing or doing something "productive." This kind of thought, that we're wasting our time, it isn't working and so on, will come up sooner or later when we're meditating.

We don't fight with these thoughts or doubts or judgments when they come up—that would be buying in and thus compounding the distraction—but just gently return the attention to the breath, over and over.

A time comes when our attention on the breath at the contact point becomes so alluring that our awareness of it becomes unbroken for periods of time.

Now, instead of having to exert energy to remain concentrated, the process seems to go on by itself. Our attention remains, for periods of time lasting from seconds to minutes, absorbed in the living sensation of the breath at a single point.

This is sometimes called "fixing" or the *preliminary sign*. It's a sign of increased concentration. This degree of concentration is sufficient to begin the practice of *insight* or *mindfulness meditation*, discussed in the next chapter. But it is possible to go further into concentration, and if we do, our insight meditation will greatly benefit because of the mind's greater deepening and ability to focus.

To go deeper into tranquillity, should we choose to do that, requires spending longer periods of time focused on our meditation. We may want to go on a meditation retreat at some point, whether privately or in a group, because it greatly increases our momentum.

When our awareness at the contact point is deep and unbroken enough for long enough, a new kind of sign will arise in our concentration. We will begin to see a light inside. This is the *nimitta* (the sign).

At first this light will be just a point of light, and it will be noticed where we've been concentrating attention—at the tip of our nose. This point of light is called sometimes the *acquired sign,* because now we've acquired something new. We continue to watch our breathing, but gradually shift attention to the point of light itself.

As we do that, the point of light gradually becomes more vivid. It can begin to look like the sun or the moon or a wisp of smoke. It can begin to spread like stars in the evening, or become a brightness that paints the inner sky.

It can also move to a different location, either inside the body in the chest or belly, or out in "front" of one's closed eyes. It is different for each person.

When we've stabilized this sign, so we can acquire it whenever we like and maintain it for as long as desired, we're said to be in *neighborhood concentration*. It's called "neighborhood" because now we've in the neighborhood of the 1st Absorption.

The Natural Way

It can be compared to the place, when driving into a city, where we pass the city limits. We're not downtown yet, but we've passed into the city.

We now direct our attention only to this stabilized inner light and hold our concentration there. As we do that, qualities of this unusual state begin to be noticed—sustained attention, extreme rapture, and bliss.

What we do now is subtly shift our attention to the qualities themselves. Our awareness of the breath and of the light remain, but they're no longer the focus. Instead we focus on these qualities of sustained attention, rapture and bliss; we "gather them in" until they are very strong and steady. We're now in the 1st Absorption.

For the practice of mindfulness meditation, this degree of concentration is more than sufficient. In fact, we can begin mindfulness meditation with no preparation in concentration at all, in what's known as starting with "bare attention."

Or we can develop concentration to the level of the preliminary sign (an unbroken awareness of the breath), neighborhood concentration (the stabilized inner light), or the 1st Absorption.

Though none of these is necessary, each increase in our concentration ability will help our mindfulness to go deeper and progress more easily.

It's also possible to go higher into the Absorptions if desired. In brief, to enter into each higher Absorption we let go of the crudest quality of the one below it. Thus to reach the 2nd from the 1st, we let go of awareness of sustained attention and focus on just rapture and bliss.

To reach the 3rd Absorption from the 2nd, we see that rapture is a gross quality compared to bliss; and so we let rapture go and focus on bliss and equanimity alone. To reach the 4th we see that bliss still has some disturbance compared to equanimity, and so we focus on the latter. And there are even higher ones.

All the absorptions are extremely profound levels of tranquillity and peace. Why then would we want to go anywhere else? Isn't that the end of the journey?

CHAPTER 22

INSIGHT

That was the question the Buddha asked himself. He had studied under the foremost meditation masters of his day and had attained all eight levels of profound absorption. Yet he was brilliant and perceptive enough to realize that he still was not truly free, that he was not truly liberated from suffering yet.

How did he realize that? He began to notice that no matter how spiritually "high" he got in the absorption levels that he still came down. He noticed that when he stopped doing these profound concentrations his normal crazy mind would come back, complete with all of its conditionings.

He noticed that while the five hindrances were completely absent while he was in the absorption levels, they were still there when he came down from his profound concentration. He was still capable of feeling ill-will or anxiety, of feeling restless or bored, of clutching at things in the world. He noticed that he was still capable of suffering. He wasn't truly free of suffering yet, and so true liberation was not yet his experience.

So he decided to try an experiment—he would go the other way. Instead of concentrating on one object, he would open his consciousness up to whatever wanted to be in his mind at the moment. But he decided to *observe* the motions of his mind rather than participating in them. And here was born the discovery of mindfulness meditation, surely one of the most momentous events in the whole history of humankind.

Mindfulness is something that we all have to some extent. Anytime we notice that something we've done has caused us suffering, anytime we notice that we're not getting the results we want, anytime we notice the rapidity with which one mind-state can change to another, we're using mindfulness.

When we're doing concentration meditation and we notice that our attention is distracted, it's mindfulness that does the noticing and then brings our attention back to the primary object.

So we all have some mindfulness. But now we want to deliberately cultivate it, like cultivating a garden, so that it becomes very powerful and steady.

The Natural Way

What the Buddha did was to begin systematically studying his mind. Not by thinking about it, but just watching it in silence. Just watching it move.

In effect, the openness of the heart towards others and the world that Jesus preached about is now brought inside and applied to our internal thought stream.

We take a step back from our thoughts and beliefs, desires and aversions, etc., and instead watch this inner thought stream with great love and acceptance. We become students of our own mind, to appreciate it and see how it works. Not by analyzing the mind or thinking about it, but by directly observing it.

What we normally do is this: We have some story or belief about somebody or something. And around that story or belief other stories and beliefs attach themselves. Now we have what's known as a "chain of thought."

This chain of thought is accompanied by an emotion, whether subtle or intense, and often a negative one. "They shouldn't have done that," goes the story, or "This world is rotten" or "John can't be trusted," or whatever. The number of possible complaints that our minds can generate is infinite.

Then what we normally do is take that chain of thought seriously and identify with it. It's not a belief, it's the "truth." We buy into the story or belief, we pick it up, we get involved with it. We think it's real, and then we act from that limited and conditioned place.

We spend most of our time believing in the truth and reality of our stories and beliefs. We look at life through the lenses of our stories and we take what we see there to be "the truth." But it's not. It's just a collection of stories that we tell about our experience of life.

In fact, as Byron Katie's work demonstrates so well, virtually any statement that we make about the world or other people can be turned around and applied to ourselves equally well or better.

If I have a belief that "Ellen is selfish when she ignores my wishes," I can turn it around to "I am selfish when I ignore Ellen's wishes," and if I look honestly I'll almost always find that the latter story is at least as true as the former.

So what we see in the other is what we ourselves are doing, although perhaps in a different form. If we say "The world is awful," we can turn it around, substitute "my thinking" for "the world," and say "My thinking is awful." If we really look, we'll find it.

When we actually begin to see this, we understand that no belief or story is true; they're just stories in the mind that affect our experience of reality and stimulate us to feel pleasure or pain.

In Katie's work, we write the mind down on paper so that we can stop it and look at it, inquire about it. When we begin mindfulness meditation, we're doing the same thing in effect, but now we're doing it in real-time.

The Natural Way

We're watching our thoughts and feelings and clingings moment-to-moment as they arise.

In effect, we do a new type of concentration meditation, where the object of concentration is continually changing—the object being the stream of thoughts and feelings in our own mind.

Here's where our development of concentration is so useful, because now we make use of that concentration to observe the moment-to-moment fluctuations of the mind itself. And the more developed our concentration, the more penetrating will be this observation of the mind's content at each moment.

Instead of "thinking our thoughts," going off on a chain of thought and taking our story seriously, we step back from it. We observe it with compassion and love, allowing it to be what it is, no longer trying to change it or improve it or deny it, but to just watch it.

And when we do that we see that each thought that arises, each desire or aversion or fear that arises has its own life cycle. It arises by itself, it stays in consciousness for a moment, and then falls away—to be immediately replaced by the next one.

We see that our thoughts and feelings and desires come on their own and go on their own if we don't get involved with them. They come and go like clouds in the sky come and go, like leaves floating down a stream come and go, if we don't interfere by giving them energy.

Pt 3—Freedom

In concentration we were like a gatekeeper, staying aware of the breath at that one point but not following it in or out. Now, in insight meditation we do something similar—we observe the fluctuations of our mind from one moment to the next without following any of them anywhere, without going downstream with them.

We stop getting involved. We observe the mind moving around in its kaleidoscope of mind-states without clinging to it as much as before. It sounds unusual at first, but we develop compassion for our own mind as we come to see its desperation and craziness, as we begin to really see its fear and clutching.

In doing this, it helps very much to have an anchor, something we can hold onto for some stability and balance while we're investigating the thought stream of our mind. This is where our concentration meditation comes in again, because we use the same awareness of the breath at one point that we used before, only this time as an anchor for watching the mind's thought stream.

The mind jumps around so much and is so compelling in its stories that it would be easy to stay lost in them without an anchor. Watching our breath at the contact point turns out to be an ideal anchor. That sensation is there all the time, always available in the present, yet involves no concepts itself.

So when we go off on a chain of thought or get distracted by something—and we notice that we've done that—we once more return our attention to the breath at the contact point. But now we add something else.

Using the breath as our anchor, we now *invite* all the distractions and hindrances and conditionings. We invite all the thoughts and feelings and attachments because we want to watch them.

Instead of holding the mind solely to one point, we do hold that point but then also welcome the mind to behave normally.

And we watch it.

CHAPTER 23

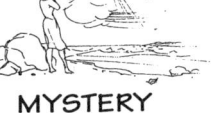
MYSTERY

Now we watch the proceedings of the mind, using our anchor as a base. We let the mind do exactly what it wants to do, because we want to observe what it normally does, how it normally behaves.

And in the very process of observing calmly without interfering, various conditionings and stories rise up out of the unconscious and take center stage at various times. We see the whole parade and just watch it without adding energy to it.

As we do so, those conditionings in our mind gradually get less vivid, less forceful. As we watch, our whole thinking-feeling-desiring-rejecting mechanism begins to gradually slow down and become less solid.

By the power of mindfulness, our conditioning, our

ways of acting out, our mind's tendency to clutch at and grab and cling and reject becomes more transparent; we see how it is. We begin to truly know ourselves.

We see that everything in Existence is in ceaseless flux, constantly changing, so that we'll always be involved in either grasping towards something we don't have or clinging to something that can't stay the same. To clearly see the mind's innate tendency to do this is to understand the basic suffering of human life.

We clearly see that impersonal energies and forces are intermingling and producing everything, and that we ourselves are the result of such impersonal interactions of energies. That is, there is no real separate self.

As we watch our mind carefully, the whole notion of "I" as something existing separately begins to weaken. We see that our sense of "I" is composed of all the thoughts that we have about ourselves—that we literally create this illusion called "I" by weaving a web of almost ceaseless thoughts about it.

In other words, we think about ourselves a lot and so create this sense of existing separately from the rest of creation. And because we have this thought-nest of ideas and feelings about ourselves, continuously being renewed in our thought stream, we sense strongly that we exist as a separate "I."

But it's all an illusion, a sleight of hand. There's nobody home. What we experience as "I" is just thoughts and feelings in our mind, like flickering images on a movie screen creating the illusion of solidity. Flickering thoughts and feelings and desires of our mind create the illusion of solid "I," of something existing separately.

Of course then, since we feel separate, we feel we have to manipulate the world in order to get what we want. And we feel suffering in doing so. Deep down, the mind feels isolated and lonely.

But as we use our mindfulness to see more clearly the impermanence, unsatisfactoriness and absence-of-self in life, a strange thing happens. We also come more and more into contact with the warm, luminous, loving intelligence at the core of us, that *is* us.

This natural essence inside is empty of all concepts and qualities, so when our minds are busy with thoughts we tend to think that it's not there. But it's always there, shining as our natural Mind. The cloud-thoughts of our thinking/desiring mind can obscure but never eliminate its luminous existence, constantly shining.

Our mindfulness gradually uncovers *that*, our true nature. But not just in meditation. Our times of sitting in meditation are really just training wheels again. We practice mindfulness in silence and solitude so that we can take it out into the world in our daily activities.

In effect, the times of sitting meditation recharge our mindfulness so that we can more powerfully use it the rest of the time, in our everyday life.

The Natural Way

Over time we develop the ability to be mindful while we're reading or shaving or conversing or working, and as we do so our mindfulness gradually begins to become more and more unbroken. After a long while it begins to go on more or less continuously, whether eating or sleeping or meditating.

People who want to go all the way to Liberation tend to retreat to solitary places, forests and monasteries and so on where they can build up their mindfulness undisturbed by interruptions, a mindfulness that can continue unbroken more and more.

As that happens the mind becomes peaceful and quiet inside. Its conditionings and stories slowly fade out of view until time itself ceases to exist and there is only the present moment, timeless and eternal. Now we see Reality without filters, because we are no longer caught in our cravings and rejections and stories about it.

Now there is only the luminous warmth and love of innate Mind, with no separate "I" there to obscure it anymore. The illusion of the separate controller/doer is gone, and now Existence itself acts through us. We move then by "intuition," by an inner and vast Intelligence moving through us and as us.

And a moment comes when it becomes clear that the mindfulness is continuous and spacious and eternal and that it will always be this way and has always been this way and is this way now in the eternal moment.

Pt 3—Freedom

In effect, time is gone, because there are no comparisons going on. Fear is gone because "Yes!" is said to everything. The state of mind is choicelessness, though Energy does move through the vessel. Feeling separate is gone because there is no one around to experience it.

This is sometimes called the "moment of maturity" or the moment of Liberation, what the Buddha called Nirvana. It's the moment when one ceases to exist—and yet continues to exist as a mind-body organism. But now this organism is transparent, available, and Intelligence moves through it, like the ocean rising in a wave.

Then this person does whatever they do. The great mystic Jacob Boehm was a cobbler by trade and remained one. Nisargadatta was a tobacco seller in Bombay and remained one. The master Ikkyu continued as a homeless wanderer, as did also the Sufi Shams-e-Tabriz. Many began to teach. Because they're no longer acting out the conditioned mind, their actions are not predictable.

One who has become Self-realized now lives in the world but not of it, as Jesus said. They create a widening ripple of love and clarity, just from their being, just from whatever interactions they have with others.

They may or may not be found feeding the poor or bathing lepers. Francis of Assisi did that. But it's impossible to say what they'll do, because there's no set model any more. They simply respond to each situation from their innate Intelligence, not knowing how or why, just

The Natural Way

doing it and noticing that their actions tend to produce greater harmony for all concerned.

Jesus was there. The great Zen masters Sosan and Dogen and Hakuin were there. So also the great Tibetan masters Padmasambhava, Milarepa, Princess Tsogyal. So were Teresa of Avila, Juan de la Cruz and Meister Eckhardt. So too the Baal Shem Tov. The great mystics Mohammed and Rabia and Hafez. Lao-Tzu. Ramana Maharshi and Osho. Byron Katie and Ammachi and many, many others from all traditions.

They awoke to their fundamental nature and that awakening transformed their little life into an expression of Life, of God showing up on earth. We humans have benefitted incomparably from those among us who have woken up to their true nature.

But we need not wait until liberation to benefit. The image of a meditator is sometimes that of a monk removed from the world, oblivious to its concerns, but meditation in everyday life contributes greatly to our own life and the world around us.

As mindfulness permeates our life more, our conditionings and clingings slowly decrease, our mind-waves gradually slow down, our actions and speech naturally express more love and generosity. Our life tends toward a natural integrity then, not from following a set of rules, but from our increasing recognition of who we are and who others are.

Pt 3—Freedom

This beneficial tendency can become especially pronounced when we consciously take our meditation into everyday activities. We use our sitting meditation each day to recharge our mindfulness, so that it can be more readily used in the rest of our life. As we do that, we find ourselves more possessed of a certain stability, a certain feeling of well-being which is not so dependent on circumstance, a feeling of greater relaxation and tranquillity in the midst of the rollercoaster of life.

We also notice that the natural warm Intelligence inside begins to be more present, and to act through us. We become more detached about the ups and downs of life—and yet, paradoxically, more alive to life too, more present and available to its richness and beauty.

We find that things tend to "happen by themselves" more, with less pushing on our part. We find that we're more willing to let things and people be as they are, and that we want to love and nurture them more. And in the light of that love, we all mature more. The world loves itself more. God shows up again on earth—in us.

As that happens, then Love begins to fall in love with Itself again. We become happy just to be who we are, where we are, how we are, feeling what we're feeling. We naturally become more loving towards the universe because we increasingly know that we're not ever separate from it.

The Natural Way

We expand, we open, we become more available to Life, to Existence however it wants to present itself. We become more available to this great Mystery that pervades us and flows through us, and through the atoms and the stars and the grass growing in the night.

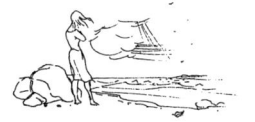

PART 4
Serenity

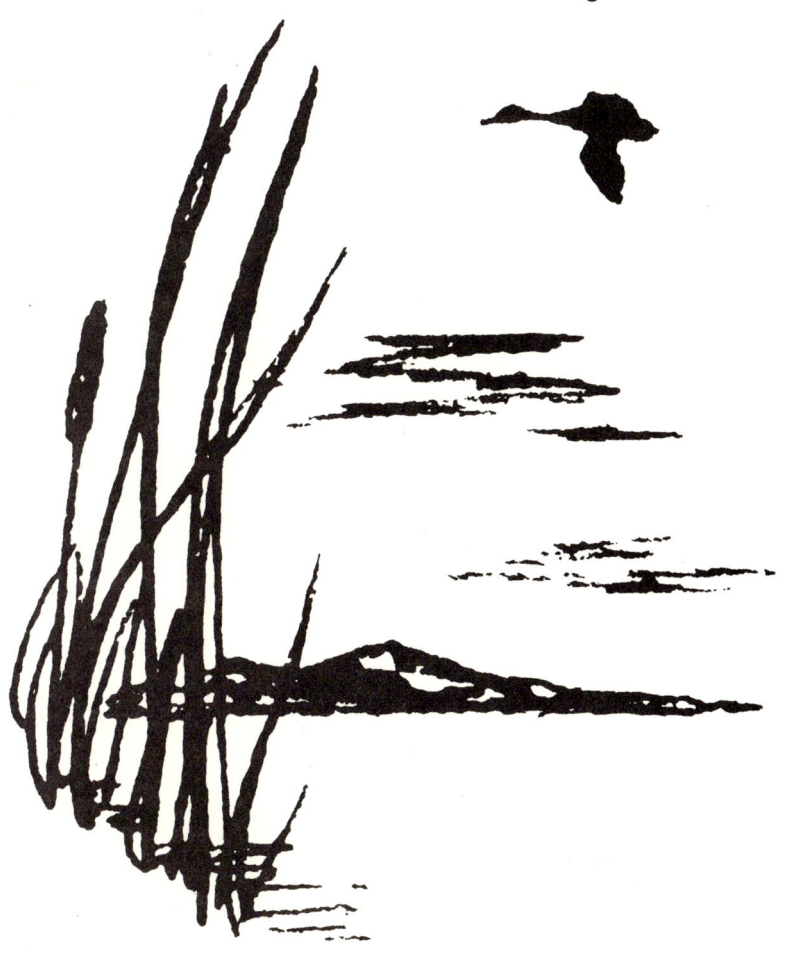

CHAPTER 24

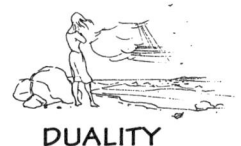
DUALITY

Now we come to the last section, which has to do with the mind, that is, how we regard the world and our role in it. In question form: What's going on here? And given the nature of things, how can I live my life in the way that's most natural and fulfilling?

Let's begin by talking about the nature of existence. For instance, all through my life I've puzzled over this question of suffering. Why does it exist? Why couldn't God have created a world without suffering?

It seems like a fair question to ask. The existence of suffering almost seems to imply that perhaps God isn't compassionate. Yet the more I've looked at that question, the more it seems that Existence can't exist except as the way it is.

The Natural Way

And what is that way? From one point of view, as an *endless series of dualities everywhere*.

For example: We enjoy having teeth with which to chew and enjoy a meal. That's "good," we enjoy being able to chew our food, it's pleasurable and nourishing. Yet that very thing, that "good" thing, also opens up the possibility of cavities and toothaches and pain in our teeth, which is "bad." But we can't have the one without opening up the possibility of the other.

Another example: We drive here and there in our car. We enjoy that, that's "good," we like being able to go places easily. Yet that very thing, that "good" thing, also opens up the possibility that we could be in a car crash and be maimed or killed, which is "bad."

In other words, I can't have the one without the other. I can't have the "good" thing without at least the possibility of the "bad" thing.

Let's say that we fall in love with someone. That's "good," it feels wonderful to be in love. Ah, the joy and ecstasy of it. And yet that person we're in love with could die suddenly, or go away for one reason or another. That's "bad"—then we'd be in despair, perhaps, and wondering why God allows such terrible misfortune to exist.

But notice that the one implies the other. The ecstasy of being in love with someone also implies the possibility of despair if we lose that person. And the more of one, the greater the potential of the other.

That is, the two potentials always exist together to the same degree and can't be separated.

So it is with the body. With this beautiful organic body we can look at a sunset or hear music or hug someone close to us.

Yet the very same body that makes possible all those "good" things is also subject to pain and illness and death, which are "bad" things.

Let's follow this out a little. Why not have bodies, then, that don't feel any pain?

Well, in fact there are a few people like that, that because of a quirk in their nervous systems don't feel any pain. And their lives are very instructive, because they tend to greatly damage themselves.

Such people can have their hand on a hot stove, for instance, and suffer third-degree burns without realizing what is happening. They tend to suffer great calamities because of their inability to feel pain.

Not feeling pain tends to quicken the deterioration and death of the organism. That is, the ability to feel pain has a much greater benefit than cost.

As Nature evolves, it produces organisms capable of feeling much greater pleasure; but with that comes the potential for additional pain, including the ability to feel emotional pain. The two have to exist together.

And that is why we humans are capable of feeling so much pain on so many levels, because we have many gifts—mental, physical, emotional, spiritual gifts which enable us to appreciate our Existence in so many ways, which enable us to feel pleasure and appreciation.

Yet it is those very same gifts which also bring in the potential for so much pain. The two are one.

Looking at these and similar examples, we begin to understand that things need to be the way they are, that what we call the "good" and "bad" are always two parts of one phenomenon. The one can't exist without the other.

When we create a mountain we create a valley at the same time. The two come into existence together. Where a front exists a back exists; they come into existence at the same time. The spinning of the planet is a single phenomenon which creates both "day" and "night."

Dualities exist together as labels. When we create the meaning and label of "hot" in our mind then we've created the meaning and label of "cold" at the same time. And then "cool" and "warm" come in.

Multiplicity comes into being in our mind, yet the underlying phenomenon is seamless and just One thing. That's how a baby experiences it. That's how an animal experiences it. They are in Oneness because they're not captured by symbolic thoughts.

And that is how we can experience it once again.

CHAPTER 25

SPACE

Let's look at another facet of duality, asking again: Can we have light without darkness?

Not really. If everything were light then light itself would have no meaning.

A candle burning in the darkness only exists as "light" because of the surrounding darkness. Though it sounds a bit strange at first, the darkness actually makes the light possible.

The very thing which we might consider useless or undesirable actually makes the "useful" possible.

To illustrate this notion the Taoist master Chuang Tzu used the following example:

Imagine, the master said, standing with both feet on the ground. Now imagine that all the ground except that which one was "using"—standing on—was cut away, so that one was standing on a small pillar thousands of feet high.

Could we go anywhere? No. When we stand on the ground, the "useless" ground that we're not using is what makes the "useful" ground—the part we're standing on—useful.

The "useless" makes the "useful" possible.

When we're in a room, it's the empty space in the room that makes the room usable and livable. If all the empty space in the room were filled up with cinder blocks then the room would be unlivable and useless.

When we enter a room, we notice the people in the room. We notice the things in the room. We notice the walls and the paintings. Our eyes are attracted to all the interesting shiny objects.

The one thing we tend not to notice is the empty space in the room, yet that is what is making everything else possible.

It's the empty space in the world—the background that we tend not to notice—that makes all the objects in the world possible and usable. Emptiness, nothingness, silence, space is the most useful thing there is.

But we tend not to notice it. Existence is filled with riotous colors of flowers and cars, with bright suns and shiny concepts and "disgusting" things too. In contrast, space isn't bright or disgusting. It's not very noticeable.

And yet it makes everything else possible. Space and form are the perfect couple.

The same is true with the internal sky.

It's the empty space in our mind, the vast and silent background of our consciousness, that makes possible all the thoughts and feelings that "we" have.

Normally we feel strongly attracted or repelled by these thoughts and feelings in our mind. We go from one thing to another, reacting and manipulating, repressing or indulging, caught in our stories.

In contrast, the space of the mind is not noticeable at first. When we just sit down in silence and do nothing for awhile, then we can begin to notice the space in the internal sky, the background of it all.

The source of all. We notice how thoughts and feelings, desires and aversions all arise and cease in this inner space. We notice how everything that arises also falls away, how every mental thing that is born also dies.

This is paralleled in the outer world, where every phenomenon that is born must also die, from stars to spiders, from civilizations to the rose on our table. Yes, even our own body must die because it was born.

Only space has no birth or death, because it is not a phenomenon. And it's undisturbed by anything that happens in it. Whether the sky is filled with dark clouds or light ones, with raindrops or sunshine, makes no difference. The sky itself remains unchanged.

The Natural Way

If we throw paint in the air, it does not color the air. Similarly, the thoughts and feelings in our mind do not affect the empty space of consciousness.

The empty space in our mind is always there, but it's subtle because it has no qualities, just like external space. Because it has no qualities, it tends not to attract attention.

But we can begin to notice it, by sitting down and listening to the silence of the mind. In that silence we can hear our own nervous system, a kind of soft high-pitched vibration, sometimes called the *shabda* or inner sound current, but even that is not it.

The real sound of silence is just deep Silence, in back of and behind everything, which we can listen to by observing our own inner thought-stream and then, as it settles down, the stillness within which it exists.

As we spend more time with this Silence, it begins to pull us, to call to us, to attract us. We sink into it more deeply. We notice the movements of the mind without getting attached to them so much, like noticing waves on a lake. As we gaze into that lake of Silence, our heart begins to see the true picture of our own face.

CHAPTER 26

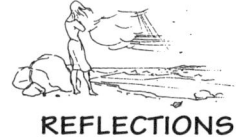
REFLECTIONS

A third aspect of duality is the duality of all our thoughts and beliefs and stories about Reality.

Byron Katie's turn-around principle advises us to look at the opposite belief when we have a judgment about someone. If I have a judgment that Bill is unkind, for instance, I turn it around to "I am unkind," and then take it inside to see if I can find it.

And the funny thing is, I always can. Maybe the cruelty is just in my mind in that instance, that I am judging Bill harshly, but it's always there. I don't know if that will be the case for you, but personally, I haven't been able to find an exception yet.

When I sincerely look in my heart, the opposite statement is always at least as true as the original one.

The Natural Way

And of course it would have to be, since we contain all things. There's the part of us that's thoughtful and the part that's thoughtless, the part that's excited and the part that's bored, and on and on.

Another example: If I have the belief that "Rosalind should care about me," I turn it around to "I should care about Rosalind," and look at that. If that's my philosophy, that people should care, then let me live it.

As Katie says, there are three kinds of business—mine, yours and God's. Who I care about is my business. Who Rosalind cares about is her business. If I have a belief that Rosalind should care about me, I'm mentally in *her* business, and I feel separate and isolated.

And how do I treat Rosalind when I have a belief that she should care, and she doesn't (or more accurately, I tell myself the story that she doesn't)? I treat her with uncaring. In other words, I'm teaching and modeling the very thing that I'm saying she shouldn't do!

And of course there's the turn-around about myself. "I should care about me." And when I look, there it always is. Perhaps I haven't been caring about myself in certain ways lately.

So let me give to myself what I'm trying to get from another. Let me be caring to myself.

But the original belief can also be turned around another way. I can write down the statement "Rosalind is uncaring" and turn it around to "Rosalind is caring."

Pt 4—Serenity

And what's fascinating is that when I look at the opposite statement inside I find it's always at least as true as the other one. Now I can see both the "uncaring" and the "caring" part of Rosalind. Both are there.

Once again I'm seeing the dual nature of Existence, which contains all things.

Recently I saw a judgment in myself about a friend, let's say his name is Sandy. And my judgment was that Sandy was insensitive, in fact one of the most insensitive people I'd ever met.

First there was the turn-around of "I'm insensitive" and it didn't take long to find that in myself. But then I did the other kind of turn-around and came up with "Sandy is sensitive." And when I looked, he was.

In fact when I really looked, it became apparent that he was one of the most sensitive people I'd ever met! He had both qualities—"sensitive" and "insensitive"—to a high degree.

Even more true is that he has neither quality. Both of them are just my stories about him, and really, neither one is true. If I truly want to be in the present with Sandy, I have to meet both stories with understanding. Can I really know that either one is true? No.

Actually, Sandy is neither sensitive nor insensitive. He just does whatever he does and I start telling stories about it. If I truly want to connect with Sandy or anyone else I have to see them without attaching to my stories about them. I have to be willing to look at that person without beliefs; then I can see him or her with love.

This dual nature of Reality extends in every direction, to every possible place. Any being that I see as "ugly" I can also see as "beautiful" if I look carefully enough. And of course they're really neither; they're just whatever they are.

Not long ago a trial of the president was going on. One side said that he lied and obstructed justice and that it was extremely reprehensible, and the other side said that even if those things were true that they didn't rise to the level of impeachable offenses.

And when I looked, I saw that they both had part of the truth. Both sides of the duality had some truth to them. And once I saw that, I could also see that neither side was really "true" in any ultimate sense. Both were just storylines.

One night I saw the PBS News Hour, anchored by Jim Lehrer. And he was interviewing two people who took opposite sides in that partisan debate.

What was interesting was that while the two partisans were passionate with the tension of advocating their positions, he was just twinkling! He was the only person there who was relaxed, because he wasn't taking sides. He was allowing both sides to have their positions without getting caught up in either one.

The Zen master Sosan comes to mind again:

"The great Way is not difficult for those who don't cherish their opinions."

The great forest master Ajahn Sumedho asks why we feel it necessary to take sides in any dispute that may come to our attention.

Why? Why the need to take a side, to have some opinion?

As soon as we take a side, we're arguing with some aspect of Reality and feeling the separation of that. Why not just let What Is be the way it is—It's going to be that way anyway—without taking sides about it? And then just doing whatever we do.

But a very interesting question arises:

If I don't take a side, how will the "right" ever be supported and prevail? And if I don't attach to beliefs or opinions, how can I ever make a choice or decision?

CHAPTER 27

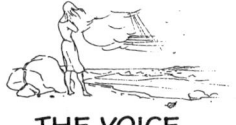

THE VOICE

This next part is a little hard to describe, but it has to do with following what can be called the inner Guide or the Voice or one's inner Intuition.

When there is a little more detachment concerning our most sacred stories, then it's as if the curtains of life part a little, allowing a little more Light in through the window. Something Vast moves through us, as us.

It's as if a kind of transparency happens, and the Melody moves through the vessel a little more easily, because it's a little more empty. The leaf flutters in the direction of the Breeze. One's little life no longer belongs to oneself so much.

Then one is just following the Intuition wherever it goes; the Energy moves by itself through the vessel. The

Pt 4—Serenity

hollow flute plays a melody. Or rather, the silent Melody plays through the flute.

To some of us that may sound a bit too out-there, so let's get practical. How do we follow our inner guide, our inner intuition?

First of all, we begin to notice the places where we're rigid, where we're holding so tightly to our beliefs, where we're worshipping at the altar of our stories. These are the ones, usually, that we hold most sacred or true, and/or the ones that we have the most anger or grief or fear or righteousness about. "They shouldn't have done what they did." "Nothing I do matters." "He/she/it doesn't care about me." "Jenny is judgmental." "This world is a screwed-up mess." And so on.

The stories that we're attached to can be political, social, economic, personal, whatever. Often we notice a lot of pain around them. The resentment or despair or anxiety or isolation that we feel always comes attached to some story or series of stories that we're clinging to.

It's not that we let the stories go exactly, but that in the very seeing of them *as* stories they begin to let go of themselves. As Katie says, we look into each story as it comes up and ask if we can really know that it's true, and see that we can't really know that. We ask who we would be if we didn't have this belief. Then we turn each belief around and see that every which way that we can turn it around is at least as true.

The Natural Way

When we begin to catch a glimpse of the inherent duality of Existence—when seen through our concepts—when we begin to see that all stories come in pairs of opposites, and that the very things we deny the most also have some truth, the let-go begins to happen by itself.

If we suddenly notice that our fist is clenched, in that very noticing the fist unclenches. It's not that we do anything; rather, we notice our fist is tightly clenched and it unclenches by itself, just from the noticing.

If we're frowning and suddenly look in a mirror, the frown will disappear by itself. We didn't realize we were tense in that way, and the very looking causes a relaxation to happen. It happens by itself.

Similarly, when we notice how tightly we're clinging to certain beliefs and stories, they begin to relax by themselves. And in that increased transparency the Energy moves by Itself.

I've noticed that there's two stages to this, which later on become one stage. The first is hearing the inner guide, and the second is honoring it.

There are many voices in our heads. How do we know which is the true inner voice, the inner guide? The simple answer is, We just do. We *do* know the difference. For one thing, It moves us. It doesn't feel like a decision, but rather like Energy moving by itself.

Second, the mind is in fear and likes to be secure. Its thoughts are about achieving greater safety, security and comfort. It is even willing to hurt others to achieve some high-minded goal. In contrast, the inner Melody tends to come from love and possibility. It comes from great love and compassion and mystery and magic.

This inner Voice is not necessarily a "voice." It can be, but it can also be a deep bodily feeling or a vision. Something moves inside that feels harmonious.

That's a sign too. When we're following the inner guide, though there may be difficulties on the surface, deep down we feel very aligned somehow.

The mind isn't always comfortable with what the inner guide suggests; sometimes the mind says this must be crazy. There's a feeling of some unpredictability, of stepping into the Unknown.

The mind can wobble, going back and forth about potential decisions. It can argue any side of anything. But the inner Voice just clearly moves when we have the courage to honor it, when we have enough transparency to let the Intelligence move by itself.

Third, the Voice has a certain excitement or sparkle about it, even though it comes from peace and stillness. It's the difference between saying "It's not bad, it's pretty good," and "I love it!" Feel the difference?

Did you ever try to remember a word? And somebody suggests one, and you go "Not really." And they suggest another and you go "Well, sort of." And then a third one, and suddenly you go "Yes! That's it!"

The Natural Way

The inner guide is similar to that. There's a feeling of rightness and alignment, especially in the body, even when difficulties are great. Sometimes it leads to places of great insecurity. One doesn't really know where one is going; it feels like a sort of confident groping.

Above all is the feeling of trust. A deep trust in existence is the ultimate cause—if there is one at all—of feeling transparent to the natural flow of things. And conversely, the more we relax and allow the movement of the inner energy the more trust we develop.

I don't wish to give the impression that I'm a master at this. I've been attempting to honor the inner guide for ten years or so, but haven't always had the courage. At times I've been aware enough to just follow it throughout the day, and other times too caught in fear or logic. But I've followed it in both "little" and "big" things often enough to know the taste of it.

About a year ago, for example, I was driving home one day about 3pm when suddenly the initial title of this book appeared as a kind of vision in my consciousness. There was a strong feeling to allow myself to sit down and just start writing on it at once.

Well, but that didn't fit in very well with my plans for the next weeks and months. And it didn't seem very practical either because it didn't appear to be money-making. But I started in anyway—I've learned to just go ahead and trust whenever I can.

Pt 4—Serenity

I could have ignored it of course, or at least there is that appearance. But if I did, I knew from past experience that things wouldn't seem as harmonious, that something would feel "off" in my body, that life would start to seem less alive, like going-through-the-motions.

Not to have followed this inner guide would have felt like denying something true inside. I had done that at times, and knew what it felt like.

But so deep is the paradox that it's also clear to me that while I was making my "choice" that it was all just Being Done. On one level It's all happening by itself, and on another level I have the feeling of choosing.

How did I know it was the inner intuition when I saw that title and felt called to start writing? The clue was a kind of obvious quality about it, that this inner sense was something natural, loving, trustable.

And of course Source is doing everything whether we "follow" It or not. It is breathing us and beating our hearts and showing up as Everything There Is and doing everything whatsoever.

Language is breaking down under these paradoxes, but you know what I mean. The more we allow ourselves to be available and open, the more we trust our heart and the universe, the more the Mystery plays the flute.

And of course It always does anyway...

CHAPTER 28

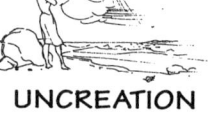

UNCREATION

Suffering seems like such a negative subject to deal with. Why bother understanding it?

Because in many ways it is the key to happiness.

Often we think that if we just get everything we want, then we'll be happy. But in fact that's not the case. Even if we had wealth and beauty beyond compare, even if we have the perfect partner and occupation, if we look closely we'll see that there's still this sense of discontent underneath, of something incomplete or unfinished.

That unsatisfactory feeling underneath pervades all human life. It comes with simply being a human being, of participating in the condition of being human.

Often we point to something in particular and say, "That's the cause of my unhappiness." We can point to our mother and father, or society, or to a co-worker or roommate, or to the "evil" in the world, or to environmental degradation or whatever, on and on and on. There is always something that we can point to as the source of our discontent.

But even if all these supposed sources of our underlying discontent were removed, even if every single thing were to magically go our way, we would still have this sense of something missing.

Why? Because that sense of discontent does not fundamentally arise from anything or anybody in the world that we can point to. It comes from within ourselves, and it comes from the very source that we've been looking to for happiness—attachment to desire.

The impulse of the mind is to desire, to cling, to attach, to want. And that, as the Buddha pointed out, is the exact source of our suffering.

Basically we have three kinds of desire. There is the desire for sensory pleasure, the desire to become somebody, and the desire to get rid of certain things.

We can all recognize the desire for sensory pleasure. We smoke, we drink, we eat, talk, get entertained, work out, on and on, to experience pleasure.

We feel that if we can accumulate enough money or vacations or the right partner or whatever, then we'll be happy. No matter what our conditions may be, the mind goes on seeking.

The Natural Way

When we tire of sensory pleasure for the moment, we turn to becoming somebody. Maybe we dedicate our life to becoming a famous actress, or to being enlightened or to having social status. And when we tire of that we want oblivion, we want to sleep for awhile. And when we wake up we want more sensory pleasure, on and on.

And there are things we want to get rid of. Certain people and situations, pain, injustice, illness, war, for openers. And when anger or fear or despair arise, we want to get rid of them too, we want them to go away. And then there's the body, which inevitably suffers aging and sickness and death.

Why? Because everything that's born has to die. All things that arise have to cease. This is something we can observe directly within ourself.

Normally when we encounter boredom or fear or whatever, we run from it. We enter the round again of eating, drinking, smoking, entertaining and so on.

But if we sit down and directly observe boredom for awhile, if we befriend it so to speak, we notice a curious thing: It goes away by itself. It ceases. And then the next feeling arises. And if we stay with that, it falls away too, to be replaced by the next thing, and the next, on and on, rising and falling, arising and ceasing.

After awhile we begin to notice directly that none of this is permanent. Our thoughts, desires, sensations, feelings all arise and fall. When we can just sit with these things as they are, neither running away nor indulging but just being with them, we notice this pervasive characteristic of impermanence. Everything both inside and outside is changing; nothing stays the same forever.

We notice that impersonal forces are acting everywhere, coming together and separating in endless variety, a ceaseless symphony of changing frequencies that meet and combine to create a "pebble" or a "person" and then separate, causing that "separate thing" to fall away. And that all of this is impersonal, just forces acting.

When we look inside at the internal parade we can't find any part of it that we can call "me" or an eternal self or the ultimate reality, because none of it endures. It all fades away; it all dies because it was born. We can't find an enduring personal "self" anywhere.

If we take apart a car looking for the "essence of car" we'll never find it; we'll just find a bunch of parts on the ground. Similarly, if we look inside for the "essence of self" we'll never find it, because there's nobody home.

The Uncreated is there, the pregnant Emptiness in the background is there, but there's no separate enduring self to be found.

The space in my room doesn't belong to me, and the space in your room doesn't belong to you. Just so, the emptiness inside you or me does not belong to "you" or "me" personally, but is the eternal silent stillness of the One, the Uncreated.

The Natural Way

As we notice that directly, we begin to see that It is acting everywhere. Did you remember to breathe while you were reading this? You didn't need to.

You and I are not so much breathing as being breathed. The Mystery is acting everywhere. You and I are meeting Ourself everywhere.

Just as when you look at your arm you don't think of it as some separate thing, but as part of you, so the rest of Existence is like that too. It's all part of You, It's all part of Itself. When you or I love, it's Existence loving Itself through the vessel of "you" or "me."

CHAPTER 29

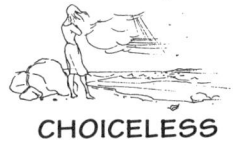

CHOICELESS

It's taken me a long time to begin to understand this next subject, so maybe I can pass it along.

We want to say "YES" to the universe, "yes" to all of Existence exactly as it is, because that's where peace of mind is found.

But if somebody asks me to dinner, does that mean I have to say "yes" to them? If somebody asks me for sex, does that mean I have to say "yes" to them? If somebody wants me to accept a business proposal, does that mean I have to say "yes" to it?

Here's the crucial thing: The "YES" we say to life is internal. It's an acceptance of everybody and everything being the way they are. In the external world, we can say "yes" or "no" to whatever is proposed.

The Natural Way

Our "yes" is to the situation being exactly the way it is, and that person being exactly the way they are, including their asking us to dinner or whatever.

And then we say "yes" or "no." And the "yes" or "no" simply appears spontaneously from within, from our inner voice or intuition.

We say "yes" to that situation and person as they are, and then we go to dinner or not. We have sex with them or not. We join in business with them or not. It's a movement from within, one that needs no justification or explanation.

But this inner Voice, this movement of energy is not a hurtful process. It comes from love and possibility. It is not interested in "breaking a few eggs to make an omelet," in Hitler's words. It is not interested in hurting or sacrificing anyone to advance some great cause. It moves from love, whether that be "yes" or "no."

"Life is internal," Katie says.

When we love Existence just as it is, it's an internal thing. Externally we can be saying "yes" or "no."

When we attach to a thought or belief that something or other is not perfection, we hurt. And that hurt is also an internal thing. It's not caused by the external event, whatever that event might be. That's just nature or somebody doing whatever they're doing.

When we hurt, it's caused by the meaning that we attach to the event or to what they did.

The external person or event may indeed have been a trigger for us, but it's our own internally-generated story about it or them that causes our pain.

That suffering is what we all share as beings. That is why the Buddha started there.

Some of us believe in God; some don't. Some of us believe in goodness; some don't. We have all kinds of different beliefs. But we all believe in pain, because we feel it. It's our common experience.

When we have a belief, like "Dad should have been wiser about money," we hurt. And it's not even true. How do we know that Dad should not have been wiser about money? Because he wasn't.

How do we know that the sun should rise this morning? It did. How do we know the world should be the way it is? Because it's that way. How do we know that being the way we are is for our highest good? Because we are that way.

How do we know that our past history is the way it should have been? Because it was that way.

Jesus and Katie and others fell in love—with it all.

The author of the Psalms in the Bible wrote this in Psalm Four:

"Lord, I praise you for that which is...
I pray for whatever you send me,
and I ask to receive it as your gift."

The Natural Way

Some of the world's great masters have talked about *choiceless awareness* and *non-interference*.

They fell in love with Existence just as it is.

Put another way, they were willing to love God the way God is.

"Love God," said Jesus, and said it was the First Commandment. But what is God?

God is whatever is in front of us. God is the person facing us, in all of their contradictory duality. God is here showing up as that person or that situation to teach us to know an aspect of ourselves.

God is the rosebush and the sewer. God is the saint and the serial killer too. People come to masters and say, "Show me God." And Jesus or Katie or St. Francis or some other great master might reply, "Show me what is not God."

CHAPTER 30

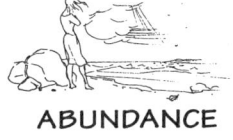

ABUNDANCE

We all seem to want abundance. Let us have abundance in our lives. Lots of whatever we want. Lots of love, romance, adventure, money, security, excitement, and on and on. An abundance of all of those and more.

But how do we get this mysterious abundance? How do we get it if we don't have it?

When I finally got it, it was pretty simple:

By recognizing that we already have it.

Where? How?

Consider this true story:

A thief broke in upon a Zen master one night. As the thief was taking this and that, the master sat quietly meditating. When the thief was almost out the door with his stolen goods, the master looked up and said, "You did

The Natural Way

not steal anything from me. I have given you these things. Thank me for them."

The thief did indeed say, "Thank you." And the master said, "You're welcome." Then the thief left.

When the thief was gone, the master gazed at the bright, silvery moon outside.

"I wish I could have given him this moon," the master said.

Abundance is recognizing that we are already abundant. And then, as a kind of side effect, we get even more abundance.

In the stillness, we know where to go and when to go and what to do. Our inner guidance tells us. Receiving and honoring that gives it All to us.

Our inner voice is guiding us all the time, if we'll hear it. It's guiding us to do the simple thing that's right in front of us, whether it's washing the dishes or making a phone call.

Whatever we're doing, we have nothing to do with it. It's all just being done. Only the Ocean Itself ever moves, moving through the wave.

"I would be what God would have me be."

That's abundance; that's sunshine.

Letting go, surrendering to the way things are. As if we have a choice!

As Byron Katie says, "How do we know it's for the highest good? Because it's here."

I have what I need. How do I know I don't need it? Because it's not here.
"I would be what God would have me be."
Can't pay the bill? Perfect.
Can pay the bill? Perfect.

Fundamentally, success and failure are stories that we tell ourselves.

"I'm worthy and successful because I have this," or "I'm unworthy and unsuccessful because I don't have that."

And the funny part is, none of those stories are true. We tell stories about how we're satisfied or not satisfied, how we're successful or not successful, and it's all in our mind.

It's all just being Done. It's a great Melody, and it's happening by Itself.

Does that mean we lie down and wait for somebody to show up at our door with a check? Not at all.

Part of the way the Melody moves is through us, as we make "decisions" and "choices," and as we listen to our Inner Guide and follow it. We can be very proactive, and yet relax and let go of the outcome. We can be active and still be in the flow of the River.

In our mind, we're as successful as our willingness to see how successful we truly are. We're unbelievably Abundant already and always. Can we see it?

The Natural Way

And beyond the duality of the mind, there is no success or failure. There's just the grace of the Mystery.

Happiness is to fulfill our destiny, our purpose.
And what is our purpose?
My purpose right now is to be drinking a cup of tea, sitting at this table and typing into a computer.
Our purpose is to be doing whatever we're doing right now. Sitting or standing or lying just as we are, with friends or without, under whatever circumstances we find ourselves—that is our purpose, that is what God would have us do.
If we're willing to be aligned with the flow of that River, we're in Abundance. It's our natural state.
And the fact is, we can't *not* be in that flow. It's just a matter of whether we're resisting it or not, relaxing or not, willing to be transparent to it or not.
And why not be willing? Things are the way they are anyway, whether we agree or not.
In the next moment, things will go to whatever's next, which may include us being very active in some way or another.
"I would be what God would have me be in this moment." Just a listening within for the Melody.
That's Abundance.

CHAPTER 31

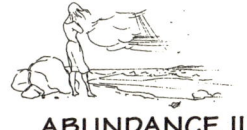
ABUNDANCE II

The fascinating thing is that the more we sink into our already-existing Abundance, the more it shows up in our life.

Whatever we pay attention to expands.

Whatever we focus on grows more real.

If we would be what God would have us be, then we just want to go wherever the Energy goes.

A great Sufi master and his followers were denied entrance to a city one rainy night. Everyone was cold, hungry and wet. The master began praising God.

One of his followers said, "Now you've gone too far. We are cold, wet, hungry—and you are praising God?"

"I can't help it," the master said. "He takes care of my needs so beautifully. Tonight I need to be cold, to-

The Natural Way

night I need to be wet and hungry. He sends me just what I need. I praise Him continually for everything. My heart overflows. This is my secret."

As Katie says, "How do I know I need it? It's here. How do I know I don't need it? It's not here. Simple."

The Melody inside then moves by Itself, in us, as us. Like a leaf floating down a stream.

And the funny part is, it does anyway. We might as well agree, because It all just is the way It is anyway.

As Rumi says,

"Do you think I know what I'm doing?
That for one breath...I belong to myself?
As much as a pen knows what it's writing."

Another factor too is that whatever frequency we vibrate at, that's what we tend to attract. Whatever kind of story we're telling, we tend to attract more energy of that kind from others. We get to live in that world.

So that the world is always a gigantic mirror for us, reflecting faithfully back to us whatever stories we have about it.

Without stories, there's no suffering.

The reality my cat Nicky lives in is very interesting. Recently he was cornered by a dog and sustained a very serious hip wound and almost died. Now he limps everywhere he goes.

But he has no story that it should be otherwise, no comparisons with what used to be. So there's no problem for him. He's limping and that's Reality, that's just the way it is. Unlike us humans, he can't generate stories and comparisons to make himself miserable about it.

The great masters wake up to that same Reality, though in a much more conscious way, without the stimulus-response of animals. They no longer worship their stories about how it all is. They just live in the Mystery, and that beautiful Mystery just moves.

The paradox is that Abundance surrounds us everywhere, like water surrounding a fish. Not only does it surround us, it is us.

Do we want to be abundant?

Become aware of our existing Abundance.

Reflect on the Abundance that we already have in our life, and that is already our nature. As we do that, we'll become aware of more Abundance in our life, and more, coming in whatever external and internal form it comes—and to tell the truth, forever already there in the first place.

It's the same principle for success or fulfillment or anything else. Recognize that It already exists, because we are as we are. We are as we're supposed to be.

Just by being here we are already success itself.

Let's celebrate it! Rather than focusing on the story of our supposed lack or failure in living up to some ideal or in reaching some high-minded goal, let's celebrate the successes that happen in our life as they come up.

If our daughter gets two B's, a C, and three D's, let's give her a celebration dinner for the B's, for what she *did* accomplish. If we finish the first chapter of a long report, let's celebrate that. And celebrate the second one when we finish that, and so on. Then we're building on a stream of successes. The momentum naturally builds.

By celebrating the abundance and success that is already there, more of it shows up. When we're choicelessly in love with however the Universe wants to present Itself, then we're already Abundant.

Abundance to Abundance.

Celebration to Celebration.

Let's celebrate our age and our situation. Let's celebrate our friends and their successes. Let's celebrate the love that exists in us already, and the little and big things we do for others already. Then more of that Love will flow through us—and then let's celebrate that too.

Let's celebrate our problems and difficulties. They are the very things that open us up, that teach empathy and compassion for others. Let's celebrate our positive feelings and our "negative" ones as well. Let's celebrate that Existence is how It is. Let's celebrate everything as the infinitely varied flowering of the All, of Ourself.

Then we become aware of overflowing gratitude. We look out at the world and wouldn't wish it to be any different than it is, even if it could be different, which it can't. We love it just as it is.

Then we feel, when we do, gratitude for all of It, even and especially our little life, knowing that it's just the way it needs to be at all moments.

Harmony. Peace.

And Love overflows from Itself to Itself through us, overflowing endlessly everywhere and forever....

CHAPTER 32

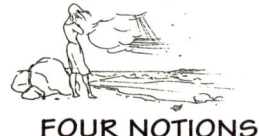

FOUR NOTIONS

About a million years ago our brains began to grow rapidly, about a cubic inch per hundred thousand years. Then the rate of growth doubled and doubled again, until our brains were growing at the incredible rate of ten cubic inches per hundred thousand years.

This great increase in brain size makes possible our symphonies and satellites and the poetry of love. All the qualities we hold dearest as human beings came about because of this rapid growth in our brain.

And what do scientists feel caused this increase in brain size? The first of several ice ages, the first ones in hundreds of millions of years. Suddenly we had to adapt to drastically different, colder circumstances.

This fueled the growth in our brain.

The hominids who lived at that time must have felt that the encroaching ice age was "bad," in that it endangered their existence. Yet it went on to lead to something that we would probably describe as very, very "good."

It was the "negative" event that made possible the "positive" event.

What is the source of our current prosperity? From one point of view, it's actually the Great Depression, which wrung out the excesses and financial bubbles of the previous cycle and re-established a solid, down-to-earth foundation for growth.

Do we really know the ultimate consequences of anything? Do we really know what is ultimately "good" or "bad," even for ourself?

We are in a deep Mystery, and that is a wonderful thing when we let go into it. Then the world evolves to whatever is next. And we get to play a part, because we're here.

Though I'm not a master at anything, perhaps I could offer here a few summations that might be helpful concerning (my understanding of) the natural way:

1. Deep, authentic Stillness.

There's no substitute, in my opinion. Allowing the mind to calm down is the essential first step—and the middle one too, and also the last—as the mind relaxes into its essential brightness and inner Knowing.

The Natural Way

Behind the stories, a Vastness with no boundaries. Dis-identification with the burden of the story that we're somebody and that we need to get somewhere.

A silent Depth from which all else flows.

This knowing deepens as we sit for a time each day, staring into that pregnant emptiness, as it were, where we slowly begin to glimpse our true face.

Also very helpful is doing The Work, undoing our stories one by one and seeing the equal truth of turning them around and applying our judgments of others to ourself. In this way our beliefs, whatever they might be, slowly detach themselves.

All clouds, whether white or black, can block the sun. And all mind-clouds of beliefs, whether "good" or "bad" ones, block the brilliant warm Intelligence of our essential nature.

"Be still and know," it says in the Hebrew Bible.

I don't know of better advice.

2. *The Melody moves from within.*

When we receive and honor that inner Voice that is there all the time, we align with Existence instantly, no matter what our circumstances.

It moves through us when we pay attention to it and don't get caught up in some story that blocks it—and when we're willing to risk going into the Unknown, risk being a leaf in the wind, risk being a holy fool.

Pt 4—Serenity

As the Taoist master Chuang Tzu said:

"Let your mind wander in simplicity,
Blend your spirit with the vastness,
Follow along with the way things are."

Let's let the Melody move through us, as it's doing already anyway! When we surrender to that....peace.

3. Fall in love with Existence as it is.
To the extent that we cease arguing with What Is, to that extent we become a hollow flute for Love to play its Song through us. We see that everything needs to be the way it is, until it changes.

We see that no one can help being the way they are. Can you help being the way you are? No. I can't either. Nobody can. It's all how it needs to be. And God is showing up everywhere as everything.

What is it that we're not willing to love yet?

What person or quality or circumstance is it that we're not willing to accept yet?

Can we see the Mystery behind all appearance?

4. Nurture Existence like a garden.
Just as a seed is perfect and yet can be nurtured by water, so too this world is perfect and yet can be nurtured by love.

The Natural Way

When we notice people's strengths and beauties and accomplishments, when we do our little part to water the seed in some area, we're part of that perfect seed evolving into Its next perfection.

We join with the flow of the River, and bask in Its silent Heart.

In closing this Part 4 on serenity, I'd like to thank a few teachers to whom I feel greatly indebted. The Buddha for his combination of compassion and deep insight. Jesus for his wide open heart and his poetic being. Osho for his great clarity. Ramana Maharshi for his beautiful silence. And Byron Katie for her remarkable compassion.

And many others—teachers, friends, loved ones who have contributed so much to me. Thank you.

I'd like to end this section with a quote from the Buddha, in the Metta Sutta:

"May all beings be at ease.
Whatever living beings there may be;
Whether they are weak or strong, omitting none,
The great or the mighty, medium, short or small,
The seen and the unseen,
Those living near and far away,
Those born and to be born—
May all beings be at ease!

Pt 4—Serenity

Let none deceive another,
Or despise any being in any state.
Let none through anger or ill will
Wish harm upon another.
Even as a mother protects with her life
Her child, her only child,
So with a boundless heart
Should one cherish all living beings;
Radiating kindness over the entire world:
Spreading upward to the skies,
And downward to the depths,
Outward and unbounded…"

Isn't that gracious and beautiful? And true?

Conclusion

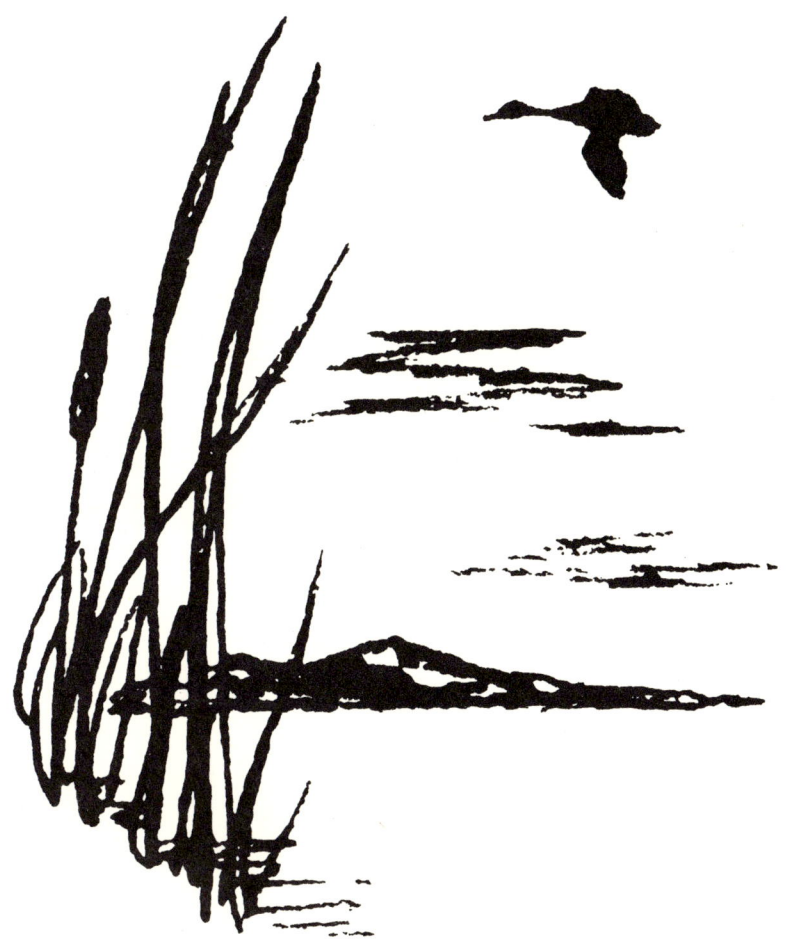

CHAPTER 33

THE NATURAL WAY

Thank you for this journey together! Let's close by looking again at some of the ways in which the natural way of things flows, like water flowing downhill.

When we go on a fast, for instance, we are literally "doing nothing"—and yet things are happening. We're trusting nature at that point; we're letting the natural intelligence inherent within us do its work unimpeded by the daily demands of digestion and activity. The results are often what we would call miraculous.

Similarly, when we move towards a plant-based or live food diet we're moving closer to the way that we ate in nature and that our bodies optimized for over so many millions of years. We're trusting nature more then; we're allowing a more natural alignment to occur between the

The Natural Way

part and the whole, between ourselves and existence. The spectacular increase in our aliveness and well-being that normally results speaks for itself.

When we eat foods that are fresh, whole, living, unprocessed—in the condition that nature made them—we are moving in a more natural way. And our bodies, which are an exquisite part of nature, respond.

This principle applies in all areas of our life.

When we see that our argument with reality is *our* argument with reality and that it has nothing to do with reality itself, we're following a more natural course, like water flowing downhill. We allow the world to be the way it is—since it's going to be that way anyway—and something inside relaxes. We're more natural.

Paradoxically, our very acceptance of the world as it is, with all its beauties and tragedies and dualities, allows us to water and nurture this perfect seed of reality in ways that we couldn't have done otherwise.

In a related sense, we're following the natural way when we undo our stories and beliefs about reality and look at it without mental filters. When we let go of the comparisons and judgments about how others should be and how we should be, we're following a more natural course. If we believe that someone is self-righteous, say, and we turn it around and see that we're really describing ourself, in that moment we see the other more naturally, that is, without our stories about them.

Conclusion

In all these areas we're moving in a more natural way, seeing and trusting that existence must be the way it is, and that this vast Way is perfect beyond measure in ways that the intellect can't know but that the heart can understand.

In a sense the whole existence is "doing nothing," happening however it does, because it's not concerned about getting somewhere else. It's already here, perfect in its present state.

In Zen they have a great metaphor for this which they call *shikan-taza*. It literally means "just sitting," and they mean for it to be taken just like that. They request that you "just sit," and they don't give any instructions about what you're supposed to do.

Okay—what could be simpler than to just sit?

But as soon as we try it we find out that we don't really know the meaning of "just sitting." What are we supposed to do? we ask. Where are we supposed to go with this? What will we get out of it?

We find out that we're doing absolutely everything except "just sitting." Even watching our mind, we find, has become a doingness. "We" are doing it. We still have an agenda. We still want something out of it all.

Even when the mind is calm, we find that we're still controlling it. We're still controlling our experience, which is what we've always been doing. We're still not just sitting. We literally have no idea how to do it.

The Natural Way

Seeing this, we try to "just sit"—and that doesn't work either. In fact, we find out that nothing at all works. Everything we do in any way to "just sit" is also part of this ever-present doingness.

We realize that we're caught in a perfect Catch-22. Everything we can even begin to imagine to get away from controlling is part of the control. The separate "I" is still very much there behind everything.

What happens then, if we're a little foolish, is we sit and sit anyway trying to "just sit." Even if we're doing other things, even if we're holding a job, we find the time to sit for a number of times each day.

And we get frustrated because we begin to deeply see the absurdity and impossibility of trying to leave the "I," the separate existence. We see that we've been trying to control everything, and that even when we try not to control everything we're still trying to control everything—and that there's absolutely no way out.

And still we go on sitting...

And this goes on for a long time...

And then, as my friend Adyashanti puts it, "Maybe, if we're really lucky, after a long time something just kind of snaps and we go a little crazy—and we find ourselves just sitting."

No agenda, nothing to get out of anything, nothing to achieve, nobody to achieve it, nowhere to go, nobody to go there. The death of the "controller."

Conclusion

Yet also, paradoxically—Life, freedom.

Now, instead of trying to control it all, we find that *It* is controlling us. In fact, It always has been. It's doing everything, and always has been. It's just that we didn't really notice.

Further, we see that It *is* us. There's no separation. So there's no need for any striving anymore. Everything is happening by itself, and it's always been that way.

We see that nothing's wrong. We're exactly where we're supposed to be. All those mistakes we made? They weren't mistakes. It was all perfect then, just as it is now. The mosaic needs both black and white stones; indeed, all the stones of every color are needed, all the events of every description are needed.

We are perfect. "You" are perfect, just as you are. It is perfect. There is nothing that needs to be changed and yet things do change. The natural way is happening by Itself. It's a living Energy, a living Intelligence.

The flower this morning. The bruise on your knee when you were ten. All the "good" and "bad" in life all had to happen exactly as it did, just as "your" life and "my" life had to happen exactly as they did.

Existence can only be the way It is. It sounds odd to say it, but It can only be the way It is. It can only exist like this, until It's different. It'll be different tomorrow, but It will still be *like this*. Just as It is. How do we know It should be this way? Because It is.

The Natural Way

Our hearts wouldn't truly open if the world weren't the way it is. It's learning to love in the face of what we call "bad" and "not right" that our hearts truly open. It's not even forgiving the world for being the way it is, but seeing that there's nothing to forgive, that it all couldn't have happened any other way than it did.

And that we can't tell the ultimate consequences of anything. The "bad" things often lead to "good" and the "good" things often lead to "bad," just as the spinning of the planet creates both "day" and "night," just as we can't create a "mountain" without creating a "valley."

In the mysterious core of silence, emptiness, "doing nothing," "just sitting," we begin to glimpse a sight of our true face. And the lines of the Zenrin come to mind:

> Sitting silently, doing nothing,
> Spring comes, and the grass grows by itself.

When we see that it's all happening by itself and that It's all as it needs to be, we begin to give the world a break and love it as it is. We begin falling in love with things as they are, including ourselves.

And we know that God shows up again on earth when *we* learn to love. If we want more love to show up in the world, let it come through us. Where can it come from except through us? "We" in the broadest sense are the only ones here—the only One here.

Conclusion

Paraphrasing Jesus, let us learn to love this world as it is in all its aspects, and ourselves and others as we are. That love and acceptance of what-is can accomplish things that nothing else can.

The world is actually one living organism—Gaia, it's sometimes called. Everything happens together and depends on everything else. Rain depends upon trees, for instance. Without trees there can be no rain. At the same time, trees depend upon rain. Without rain there are no trees. It's one system, trees and rain together.

In a similar way, life has altered its environment—temperature, gases in the air, etc.—to make it possible for life to continue. Life has adapted to the environment and the environment has adapted to life—they're one system, one thing. *The One*.

We don't exist separately from other life. We don't exist separately from the environment or separately from each other. We don't exist separately.

In "just sitting" with the stories and fears and joys of our life, we come to see that it's not "our" life. *It* has life, as you and me and the dogwood tree.

Then instead of trying to control things, we see that *It* controls us, *It* moves through us, It *is* us. The Mystery moves in us. We do whatever we do, but from a place of "doing nothing," because we're not trying to get somewhere with it. We just follow the natural way, like water flowing downstream, and feel gratitude.

The Natural Way

This natural way flows by itself, like water. When we "do nothing" on a bodily level, when we rest and fast and trust that the organism knows what it's doing, the vital power in the organism heals itself to the greatest extent possible. It's the very "doing nothing" that allows the body to heal itself, to regenerate.

On a planetary level, we may find ourselves willing someday to do a kind of "fast"—a voluntary, planet-wide lowering for a time of most production and consumption activity—to allow Gaia to heal itself of its accumulated pollution and toxemia.

"Doing nothing" is also what we do when we fall in love with the world. We're no longer asking the world to be different or better somehow to fit our ideas of how it's supposed to be. We're just willing for it to be how it is while we do whatever we do.

We see our stories and beliefs without needing to get involved, just as the ocean is not concerned by fish swimming in the sea. And if feelings of fear or irritation or sadness arise in us, we give them the same compassion that a mother would give to her child.

We're following the natural way when we take the time to appreciate the world, to see what a miracle it is, to feel gratitude for our part in the play. We're following the natural way when we release our agenda and who we think we are and just follow the inner guide wherever it goes, letting the great Mystery unfold.

Conclusion

Then we sing and dance and play within, knowing that It will all turn out okay because It already did.

Then the Energy moves us, just as It's breathing us and beating our heart and filling our heart and swaying the leaves and moving the stars.

We follow that loving guide inside that aligns us to the flow of Existence—or rather, to the knowledge that we and everything else are already aligned.

How do we follow it? How do we hear it?

"We" can't, of course. Because it's the Intelligence itself that always moves.

Yet we can "follow" It in a sense by willingness, by a deep surrender and listening of the heart as the Energy of gratitude moves through us.

We "follow" It too by being willing to see that the Melody is already playing always, everywhere, endlessly, and especially in our own heart.

To the beauty that is you... May you experience much kindness and serenity until we meet again.

Love,

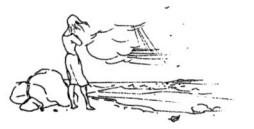

James Sloman is an investigative writer whose subject is the human condition. He has sought understanding from a wide range of great teachers past and present, famous and obscure, and traditions ranging from India to the kitchen table.

Originally trained in philosophy at Princeton and with an MFA in film from Columbia, he draws from experience in an eclectic career which has included being a copywriter, assistant editor and computer programmer in New York, a novelist in rural Massachusetts, a trader in Chicago and a market theorist in San Diego.

In addition to presenting occasional courses on theories of financial markets, Jimmy has spent over two decades teaching seminars and workshops on the natural way, including spirituality, consciousness in everyday life, nutrition, discovering our true calling and accessing our inner guidance.

He lives near San Francisco.

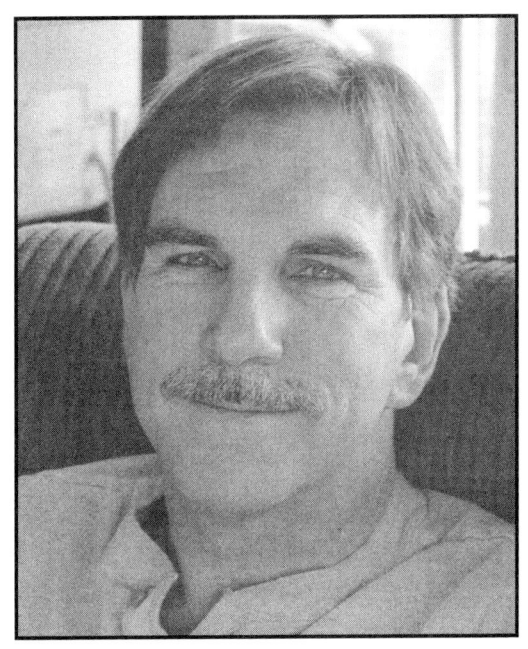

Thank you for reading
The Natural Way.
If you liked it, please tell
your friends about it.

Products by James Sloman,
available from OceanBlue
Publishing, include:

The Natural Way
Nothing
Handbook for Humans
The Ripple
Affecting Our Reality
Songs From The Bottom Of The Sea

Descriptions are on the next pages.

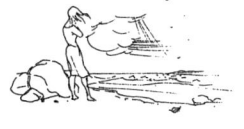

To place an order:

Call: 800-838-7360

Abroad: (707) 838-6200

Or mail the order form
in back to:

OceanBlue Publishing
98 Main Street
Tiburon, CA 94920

www.ocean-blue.com

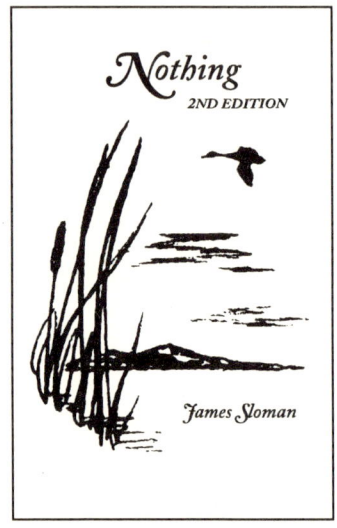

NOTHING
Uncovering Our True Nature
2nd edition, 200 pages, $14

What is our true nature? And how do we access it? How do we glimpse it? A facial mirror will do for our face, but what about the mind itself?

Nothing is a mind-mirror which holds up a glass to the mind so that we can begin to observe it. And in that looking, an opening can occur in which life is seen as inherently gracious and rewarding.

In this revised 2nd edition of *Nothing*, investigative writer James Sloman takes us on a journey through the mind and the context in which it resides. In the process, he clearly and precisely demystifies the essence of the mind so that our true Nature can be revealed. He skillfully and playfully uses stories, quotes and fables from many paths and traditions to assist in uncovering our inherent bright, warm and loving Nature.

In reading *Nothing* the eye is pleased as well as the soul through simple, beautiful and elegant illustrations by the noted artist Tonia Weeks. *Nothing* was awarded The Design Award of the Printers of the Carolinas.

True unsolicited comments from readers:

"I was truly moved and changed by reading this book. I have been on the path for a number of years reading all kinds of books, and *Nothing* is the best...truly beyond words."
—*JLS, Utah*

"I have read *Nothing* several times now and think it is the best book of its type that I have ever read."
—*EW, New Jersey*

"I get great pleasure from *Nothing*. I open it often to remind myself of the truths therein."
—*VB, Chicago*

"*Nothing* is the best book I've read in a long time...a beautiful job."
—*SG, Phoenix*

"*Nothing* came as we were experiencing an unusually tough situation...it helped immensely."
—*J&PS, Miami*

"I have read extensively in this area but had not previously encountered a work wherein clarity of vision and uncluttered sensibility were so evenly balanced... *Nothing* speaks straight to the heart...it's helping so much."
—*VL, N. Carolina*

HANDBOOK FOR HUMANS

A Comprehensive Synthesis of Paths to Personal Growth
560 pages, $24

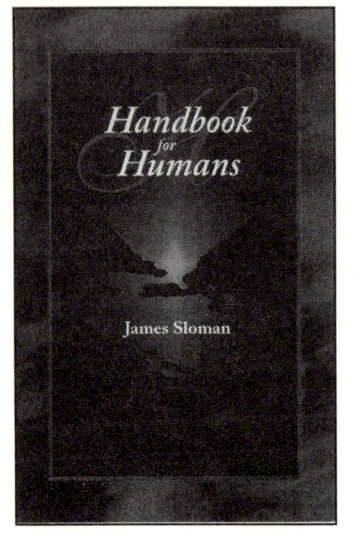

We get handbooks when we buy appliances and cars—why not one on basic information for living?

"A wonderful new book by Jimmy Sloman is the manual he wishes he had received when he was growing up. *Handbook for Humans* is the culmination of a lifetime of learning and eight years of writing. In it, the author distills the wisdom of dozens of traditional paths to health, happiness, success and peace into an easy-to-digest overview of how our lives really work. *Handbook for Humans* succeeds as an excellent guide to help us achieve balance, equanimity, vibrancy and wholeness in our lives. We recommend it highly."
—Patti Breitman, *EarthSave Marin*

Handbook for Humans is actually a collection of four books in one cover, addressing the *Spirit, Mind, Heart* and *Body*. Each of these dimensions is then divided into an inner and outer area, allowing the reader to clearly grasp the inner work that will support the expressions he or she would like to take into the world.

"If there were only one book you could read to navigate your way on the path of life, *Handbook for Humans* would be the perfect choice. Jimmy Sloman has created a treasure trove of wisdom...that feeds the soul and body. I am grateful for this book."

—Susan Smith Jones, author of
Choose to Live Each Day Fully

Peppered with dozens of real-life stories along with fables, folk tales, quotes & studies, *Handbook for Humans* is the manual many have been looking for to use in daily life as a course in what works.

"...I complimented James Sloman on his skill in integrating ideas from many spiritual sources in his book *Handbook for Humans*. Sloman is known in financial circles for his work on the Delta Phenomenon and Adam Theory..He started a book on markets more than eight years ago but put it aside when he felt directed to prepare the *Handbook*. (He didn't know writing it would take so long), but readers will not be surprised because his book is so thoroughly researched, from Taoism to diets, from evolution to empathy..."

—Vern Barnett, *Kansas City Star*

THE NATURAL WAY
An Inquiry Into Happiness
232 pages, $14

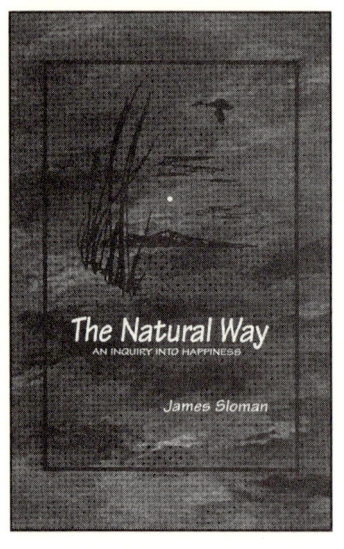

The Natural Way explores the connection between happiness and what Lao-Tzu called "the natural way" of things—and how it might apply in various aspects of our life.

The Natural Way shares many stories, insights, studies and examples from a number of great traditions.

The book has four parts:

Happiness is about opening the heart and falling in love with the world.

Vitality is about honoring the body's healing wisdom in unfolding our natural well-being.

Freedom explores the inner journey in ways that are practical and down-to-earth.

Serenity talks about following our inner knowing, our inner guide.

The emphasis of all four parts of *The Natural Way* is the uncovering of the warm, bright, loving intelligence within each of us.

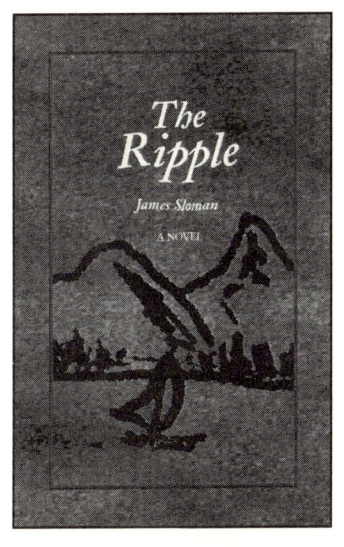

THE RIPPLE
A Mystery Story
Of A Being's Journey
A novel, 400 pages, $15

"*The Ripple*, by James Sloman, shows the broad range of Mr. Sloman's prodigious talent. Set in the overpowering environment of New York City in the 70's (when it was written), *The Ripple* chronicles the breakdown of the human psyche as it strives for autonomy and recognition against the metropolis' spiraling whirlpool of anonymity and powerlessness.

"Sloman creates a darkly tragic yet humorous world where rage and regret dance a tango of bittersweet promise resigned to inevitable defeat. Punkin Miller, a computer programmer who is tormented by fellow workers, shop keepers and women beyond his means, reaches a breaking point...The result is a horrific, heartbreaking and mesmerizing ride as the reader follows Punkin Miller through the maze of mental meltdown, cat and mouse intrigue, and finally, total surrender to the crashing permanence of fate.

"There are many valuable lessons to be learned from *The Ripple* about the human condition. But make no mistake. *The Ripple* is a dark journey through the underside of the beast, and though redemption is found at last, the price is the loss of a soul."
—Michael Gottlieb, author of *Squeeze Play*

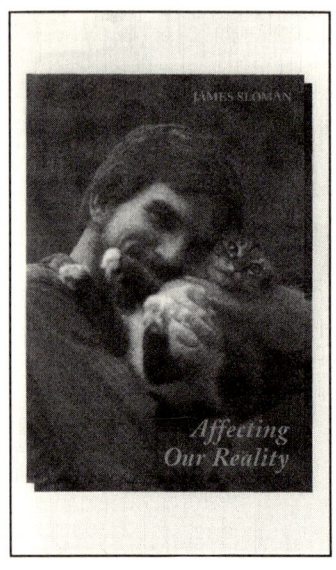

AFFECTING OUR REALITY
Chicago Talk Series
Set of 4 cassettes, $22

Topics of Discussion:

- Finding your calling in life
- The role of play in vision
- Looking at what's real
- Loving, accepting ourselves
- Surrender and freedom
- The paradox of feelings
- Everything as a gift
- Life as mystery and magic

"A kind and soothing voice...I felt a sense of self-awareness, a warmth, a glow, a knowledge I've known before only I don't know where...a real insight to life and living."
—S.K., Miami, FL

"Thank you...wonderful!"
—J.M., St. Louis, MO

"So good...excellent!"
—C.C., Monterey, CA

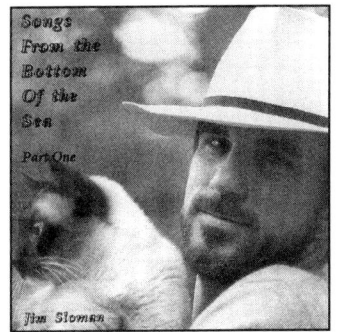

SONGS FROM THE BOTTOM OF THE SEA
18 songs, voice & guitar
Set of 2 CDs, $22

"Jackpot!"

"Now, perhaps more than ever, it seems that you can't swing a Martin steel-string without hitting a folk singer. But one of the great things about the persistence and popularity of singer-songwriter types is that every so often a new voice comes along that reminds us that folk singers can still be legit and likeable even in the '90s.

"In the vast sea of singer/songwriters, Sloman's rich, clear, well-recorded voice stands out...

"There's plenty here for folkies and non-folk fans alike to grab. In addition to his use of abundantly vivid personal details and storytelling and songwriting tactics ("Charlie"), Sloman's most surprising trick could be his rewrites of cover songs like "The Night They Drove Old Dixie Down" or "Summertime," where he gets the words down right but embellishes and distends the music, adding his own melody underneath to create a completely new song that's respectful and appreciative of the original, but fresh and vital nonetheless."

—*CMJ New Music Report*

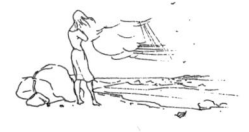

To place an order:

Call: 800-838-7360

Abroad: 707-838-6200

Or mail the order form with your check to OceanBlue Publishing

---

*SHIPPING & HANDLING

In the US, add $4 shipping for first item, $1 for each additional item. Express and international, please call for shipping.

www.ocean-blue.com

OceanBlue Publishing
98 Main Street
Tiburon, CA 94920

ITEM	QTY	PRICE	AMOUNT
The Natural Way		$14	
Nothing		$14	
Handbook for Humans		$24	
The Ripple		$15	
Affecting Our Reality set		$22	
Songs From....Sea set		$22	
Subtotal			
CA residents add 7.5% tax			
Shipping*			
Total Enclosed			

Name _____

Address _____

CityStateZip _____

Phone or e-mail _____

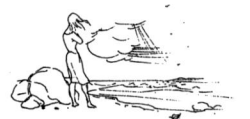